Breakthrough Therapies:

Crystal Acupuncture[sm] & Teragram[sm] Therapy

Margaret Rogers Van Coops,
Ph.D. DCH(IM)

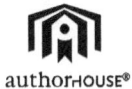

authorHOUSE®

AuthorHouse™
1663 Liberty Drive
Bloomington, IN 47403
www.authorhouse.com
Phone: 1-800-839-8640

First published by AuthorHouse   6/16/2011

ISBN: 978-1-4184-4864-6 (sc)
ISBN: 978-1-4184-5829-4 (e)

Library of Congress Control Number: 2003099846

Printed in the United States of America

TABLE OF CONTENTS

ACKNOWLEDGEMENTS

I offer my acknowledgement and appreciation to all those clients who came to me in trust and allowed me to expand and improve my healing skills with Crystal Acupuncture^{sm} and Teragram^{sm} Therapies. These therapies were done with a two-fold objective: that the clients might recover and that the therapies really would work. And so it happened!

I dedicate this book to my husband, Stephen Van Coops, whose constant belief; support and guidance of me in the USA helped me to achieve my many successes.

I acknowledge my Spirit Guides who, in my time of suffering, opened the doors of my awareness into the manifestation of these therapies.

Thank you everyone…

Dr. Margaret

PREFACE

Crystal Acupuncture^sm evolved over the years because of various ailments I manifested that required treatment. I inherited Parkinson's Disease, a major illness for which there was no cure. My quest for finding the right stones to heal myself opened up my journey of discovery. I carefully selected the stones, now called crystals, and my Spirit Guide, Master Chang, taught me the techniques I ultimately developed.

Teragram^sm Therapy began in a very unusual way. I was already deeply involved in my research on Crystal Acupuncture^sm at the time and was ready to promote it. My first task was to find a wholesaler who could keep me supplied with the crystal points that I had chosen. Hence, my visit to Fred Miller who, at that time, was busy making Agate clocks.

During my negotiations with him, I kept being drawn to large Agate slices that his daughter was working on. I watched her carefully sticking the clock numerals on each slice and then placing the hands in position as she attached the clock workings behind. The more I watched her, the more I realized that it was not her clock-making that intrigued me, but rather the Agate slices themselves.

After having carefully selected certain crystals for my Crystal Acupuncture^sm sets, I asked Fred about the Agate slices. He gave me one to hold while he explained how they had been cut and chemically colored. The slice I held was very heavy, being eight inches in diameter and a quarter inch thick. I was fascinated by the many colors that radiated energy towards me. I felt like a child with a new toy. I didn't know why, but knew I had to have a few of them. So I asked him to sell some to me. He insisted on giving me eight slices of various colors. They were red, blue, green, yellow, purple and pink as well as two others that were multicolored. Together they weighed approximately five pounds.

Back home, I studied them. My Spirit Guides had been with me the whole time I had been talking to Fred, but they had said nothing. Now, alone with me, they spoke and confirmed to me that I had a new therapy to begin investigating.

My first step was to use them on myself. As soon as circumstances allowed, I found a quiet time to lie down and placed six of the heavy Agate slices on my Chakras. In no time at all, I was experiencing swirling energy in all of my Chakras and a shifting of my Five Bodies. I knew then that this was truly the beginning of a new adventure for me. During my final research, I chose the name Teragram^{sm} Therapy. Within the word Teragram are anagrams. *Terra* is of the Earth. *Gram* is a weight and then, of course, *Agate* are all included. It also is my name spelled backwards. Great! My secret mark!

Over the years, I discovered just how effective and important Agate is as a healing stone. When I combined Teragram^{sm} Therapy with Crystal Acupuncture^{sm}, I found my clients recovering from their illnesses at a much faster rate. Many of my clients volunteered to be my guinea pigs and I owe much to them for their trust and support in allowing me to experiment.

Since then, I have taught and trained individuals in America, England and Japan to practice Crystal Acupuncture^{sm} and Teragram^{sm} Therapy. These Therapists are happy to report to me from time to time and the response is always the same: "The clients are recovering quickly and are emotionally and mentally calmer and happier."

Crystal Acupuncture^{sm} and Teragram^{sm} Therapy are effective in conjunction with any traditional medical treatment as well as with any alternative medicine and therapy. These therapies are non-invasive and have no bad side effects. In the pages to come, I intend to help you, the reader, make up your own mind about using Crystal Acupuncture^{sm} and Teragram^{sm} Therapy.

I strongly recommend that you also purchase and make ample use of my illustrated book, *The Book of Crystal Acupuncture^sm and Teragram^sm Therapy Diagrams*, which provides numerous detailed diagrams and directions for use of the stones described here. Treatments of specific disorders and conditions are described in that book. **Margaret Rogers Van Coops'** *Breakthrough Therapies: Crystal Acupuncture^sm and Teragram^sm Therapy* will be of great value to those who do healing with their own collections of crystals or who purchase our packaged therapy kits.

Terms Used In This Book

Acu Points: Miniature rotating vortices of energy located along the body's meridians

Aura: A swirling mass of colors created by energy emanating from the Five Bodies. It reflects the condition of the bodies.

Base (Root) Chakra 7th (Lower Self) Major Chakra: Energy center located between the legs over the front and rear passages. Unlearned lessons are stored here.

Body Syndromes: Negative conditions affecting the Physical Body caused by blocks in the Etheric Body.

Cellular Neuro-muscular Memory: Genetic information stored at the cellular level from past experiences in this and previous incarnations.

Chakra: A vortex of energy created by many minor vortices within. Chakras are cone shaped and they stimulate growth and body function.

Clairvoyance: The psychic sense of sight (insight).

Conscious Mind: The part of the mind that deals with immediate perception and judgment. It is often mistaken and inaccurate.

Crown Chakra 1st (Lower Self) Major Chakra: Energy center located at the top of the head. It controls the neural paths of the brain and modulates energy flow in all Five Bodies.

Deep Subconscious (Spirit) Mind: The part of the mind that has direct connection with Universal knowledge and previous incarnations and can impart only truth.

Dowsing: Technique of discovering energy emanations with use of pendulums, divining rods, or other devices.

Emotional Intellectuals: Psychological model describing those who attune with their brain before they attune with their heart. They think before they feel.

Emotional Physicals: Psychological model describing those who attune with the heart before the brain. They feel first and think afterwards.

Etheric Body: Layer of emotional energy that envelops the physical body and normally protrudes about 2-4 inches away from the physical form.

Five Bodies: Five major forms that generally define our identity and purpose. They include the Physical, Etheric, Spirit, Higher Mind and Soul Bodies.

Heart Chakra 4th (Lower Self) Major Chakra: This energy center lies over the heart with its center at the sternum. True feelings are assimilated here. Positive and negative emotions generate here.

Higher Self: Another term for Spirit Body where true thoughts and emotions manifest on all levels.

Higher Self Chakras (7): Numbering of Chakras is reversed: Base is #1 to Crown #7 plus the additional 5 Cosmic Chakras that connect divine consciousness from God into awareness.

Kundalini: In India, China and Japan cultures, this is the "Chi" or electro-magnetic energy that flows upward from the Root Chakra to the Crown Chakra.

Laws of Karma: Five basic universal guidelines that assist our relationship with principles of cause and effect.

Masculine/Feminine Self: Aspects of our being generally described as right and left sides of our body. Right is masculine governing earthly existence and use of time. Left is feminine governing emotions and spiritual consciousness.

Medium: In Spiritualism, it is believed that contact with the "other side" is made through intermediaries called "mediums."

Meridian: In Oriental medicine, the meridians are the defined pathways through which electro-magnetic energies flow. There are 12 major meridians & 8 supportive meridians flowing from head to foot and back.

(Higher) Mind Body: One of the Five Bodies. This is most subtle Body, which taps Universal Consciousness and uses pure thought as an energy form.

Mini Chakras: See Acu Points. These terms are interchangeable.

Minor Chakras: Chakras located in the palms, elbows, knees and feet.

Physical Body: One of the Five Bodies. This is the densest and the one we are most familiar with through our earthly senses.

Psychometry: The psychic sense of smell and touch. We "get feelings" through this sense.

Rejection Syndrome: Dr. Margaret's description of our rejection of our own talents, skills and beliefs through childhood negative conditioning.

Solar Plexus Chakra 5th (Lower Self) Major Chakra: The largest Chakra covers the area between the navel and breastbone. Energy is absorbed and expelled here as human contact and dialog occur.

Soul Body: One of the Five Bodies. The most refined energy form is here. It defines the momentum of our growth in the Oneness and provides our link to The Source.

Soul Structure: Coding assigned to each individual giving them unique personality and focus in their life's pathway.

Spirit Body: One of the Five Bodies. Not of the Earth, this body expands and contracts according to its interaction with the lower bodies. It is replenished only by the Higher Mind and Soul energies.

Spirit Guides: Higher Ascended Soul fragments that have no incarnate form. These communicate with us as Angels, teachers and motivators. They help lower fragments to ascend to The Oneness.

Spleen Chakra 6th (Lower Self) Major Chakra: This lies just under the left rear of the ribcage and extends diagonally through the body to just under the right front ribs. It stimulates or retards the flow of energy to each of the Five Bodies.

Stages of Loss: Changes of attitude that take place when erasing personal history that causes body syndromes.

Subconscious Mind: The largest part of our mind. It stores positive and negative message units from this incarnation and controls our ability to think and do.

Third Eye Chakra (Brow) 2nd (Lower Self) Major Chakra: Located at the center of the forehead, this is the focal tool for our inner vision or clairvoyance.

Throat Chakra 3rd (Lower Self) Major Chakra: Lies over the Larynx and Thyroid gland. It balances all that is thought or spoken.

Universal Consciousness: The "God Consciousness" that encompasses the totality of all that is. We draw from this consciousness with all of our physical, mental and spiritual faculties. It is the source of all knowledge and wisdom.

CHAPTER 1

Discovering Lost Knowledge

Our Ancestors Had a Secret

Agate is all over the world. It varies in color from white to dark brown or black. For as long as we can remember, it has been used for furnishings and jewelry. Early Egyptians used Agate slabs to cover their sacred altars. Craftsmen made fine amulets of Agate and people wore them around the neck to keep themselves safe from harm. Everyone knew that Agate was a holy stone and that it protected users from evil. Thus, they believed they were closer to the Gods. History reveals that ancient cultures respected this stone, yet they were not geologists. They performed no scientific studies, so how then did those ancient ancestors of ours know so much about Agate?

The best sources for answers were my Spirit Guides, who taught me that in those ancient days, people were highly receptive to feeling emanations from everything they touched. They were Psychometrists. Psychometry is the psychic sense of touch which, in reality, is our Spirit's own sense of feeling.

Because everyone is a spirit living within a body, each of us is capable of using Psychometry. In modern times, we generally use Psychometry to sense unrest in relationships and business affairs. A few use their psychic skills to attune to their environment and the beauty of this Earth that surrounds them. It is only in the past few years that interest has grown, once again, in the use of crystals as healing tools.

Using Clairvoyance, my Spirit Guides showed me in a vision how a temple priest would prostrate himself upon an Agate altar in the hope of receiving a command from the gods. He then took the message to the people of his village. I saw how the Agate altar affected the priest's body. His Aura shifted, pulling in as though shrinking and then expanding, as negativity and fear left his body in the form of red, blue and green explosions. His mind emptied and his spirit awakened to his innermost senses. His Aura expanded and took on a golden hue. In this state, I watched as he touched his Spirit Guides and made connections. I saw his Spirit Guides join with him and, as he received their messages, his Aura changed again to a light blue. I knew he had become enlightened. I watched as dark and dull colors surfaced in his Aura and then dissipated as new lighter and brighter colors took their place. Within these colors, I could see a spectacular display of color discharges as his body relaxed. I watched as all his energies began to flow and a general healing occurred.

Once the priest had received his message of insight, he left the altar and returned to the people, appearing rejuvenated. His Aura was stronger and his life forces brighter. I watched as the priest's followers, using Psychometry, felt this change in him and placed their trust in him by honoring his words and following his commands.

The priest then gave out Agate amulets to bless the people in their times of trouble. I knew that the wearer could feel his own energy improving. He became more positive about his situation and felt more empowered to deal with his problems. My Spirit Guides told me that peoples' recoveries were most often credited to the priest and the power of the amulet, rather than to their own efforts in overcoming their traumas.

Finding Lost Truths!

"What was it," I wondered, "that the Agate table really did for the priest?"

The Teragrams made it possible for me to enter a new research phase. It

2

took me six years to learn the truth. I was already acquainted with the use of Agate Crystals and related family stones in my research. Had I not already completed this work, it might have taken me much longer. Because you, the reader, need to walk slowly with me through the process, I will go back to the beginning.

The Beginning

When I was very young, my parents used to take me to Brighton in Sussex, England where my Grandparents lived. We spent a great deal of time on the beaches there. Large round pebbles were everywhere, some too big for me to lift. As I played among these stones, I noticed that some of them seemed to emanate colors. I was particularly attracted to smaller pebbles that emitted rainbow colors. Often, I would collect a bucket-full to take home, only to find my parents insisting on my putting them back under the pretext that they belonged on the beach. I was often miserable on the way home; having been denied my stones. By the time I was nine, they allowed me to keep a few. The stones sat on a shelf in my bedroom as if waiting for me to do something with them. They were my treasures.

I learned to accept my healing powers, although I didn't understand how it happened. I knew that I grew hot and that, when I sat on a person's lap, their auras changed. When done, bright colors emanated from their heads, telling me I could get down and continue playing my games. Within moments I was picked up again and would then watch the whole procedure all over again. I didn't mind. I liked all the attention they gave me. As young as I was, I knew that healing energy was made of wonderful colors that cascaded around a person. The colors were very similar to those of the pebbles I had collected.

One day, my mother's cousin came to visit. She was visibly tired and looked unwell. She told my mother that she had a migraine. I was about to go and sit on her lap, when my Spirit Guide's voice told me to get one of my pebbles. Without hesitation, I brought it and placed it on "auntie's" head.

"What's she doing?" She exclaimed.
My mother, who was used to my little antics, simply smiled and said. "Humor her. She likes to play Doctors and Nurses!"

The adults carried on talking. Auntie complained about her life. I listened with interest when suddenly; I noticed that the stone I held to her head was pulsating. It seemed to glow with a red light and then an explosion of energy burst from it and disappeared. I was stunned. At the same time, Auntie looked at me and then at my mother.

"What did she do? My headache is gone."

"The stone did it," I said matter-of–factly.

I was consciously surprised, but inwardly, there was a special knowing. My treasure was special.

Over the years that followed, I collected many stones. My first important discovery was Quartz. I attended an 'Ideal Home Exhibition' in London. A man held a piece of Quartz out to the crowd and proclaimed that this was special. Inside every watch that he was selling, was a piece of Quartz just like the one he was holding. I was not interested in his watches, but the Quartz fascinated me. As he moved it around, I could see rainbow traces of colors from where it had been. He was waving it around and I watched fascinated by the traces it made in empty space.

When his demonstration was over, I asked him for the crystal. He told me to get lost, but he didn't get rid of me that easily. I pestered him all day, and as it was the last day of the event, he finally gave it to me to get rid of me. I thanked him profusely, babbling about the emanations of the stone. I'm sure he thought I was quite insane.

My child-like experiments were mostly carried out on my best friends. They let me poke and prod them with the Quartz stone. They gave me feedback about how it felt, which was mostly hot and tingly. I owe much to them for their indulgence. My Spirit Guides often gave me tidbits of information. I learned that Quartz was an energizer. It was receptive to my energy. I saw that I could put my healing energy into it and that it changed my energy into a laser light the spurted out at the point. When I put the point on myself, I felt my energy being amplified and was aware of energy moving inside myself. Sometimes it felt like ants crawling over me, while others times it felt like water running over my skin. Inwardly, it felt tingly and prickly. I knew I had a very important healing tool.

My discoveries about Quartz led me to test my other stones, for all of which, I had no knowledge of geology. I found that they had similar properties, which mystified me. Some stones seemed gentler or subtler in their effect.

It was around this time, that I began to learn about the existence of the other four bodies that surrounded the Physical Body. I was mystified to find that no one else seemed able to see what I was seeing. I tried showing others; some could feel the stone's effects, but most just laughed.

Discouraging Words Can Harm!

Had it not been for my Spirit Guides, I might have given up my research. I was fed up with being different. I wanted to fit in. Be like others. Have a life! Ever since I could remember, I wanted to be a nurse. Now that my schooling was behind me, I was happy to join a nursing school, The Royal Surrey County Hospital, to do my training. My knowledge of anatomy was already significant, but here I learned more. I watched medical procedures and experienced fascinating psychic visions during the processes. I saw fear, pain, anger, guilt and more in all my patients as they went through their healing processes. I knew ahead of time, those who would die from those who would recover. I saw gaping wounds and unhealthy auras. I saw weeping men and dominant women break down their energies to be reborn — their energies renewed. Every patient I touched was a healing experience for me. My Spirit Guides walked beside me daily. I was overworked and underpaid, but I was happy. I was learning so much. Then, one horrible day, the door slammed in my face.

An old lady, not quite right in the head, was due for surgery that day. Another patient gave her a glass of orange juice. I was accused of having done the bad deed. Despite my insistence on being innocent and the eventual confession of the perpetrator, it was suggested to me that I should give up the nursing profession, because I was not "subservient enough" to my superiors. Broken hearted, I returned home with the idea of entering another hospital. It never happened.

Learning to Follow the Rules

Soon after my leaving the hospital, I married and had two children. During those years, I did not do any healing with crystals. My husband had forbidden this kind of work. He'd been a preacher but had turned his back on God after his horrendous divorce. He didn't believe a true God would let one suffer so much. Of course, he did not believe in psychic things either. Instead, he introduced me to his friends who were Psychologists. To them everything in life was logically explained. I learned how to counsel the mentally insane during this period. My Spirit Guides were always close, but never interfered.

During those years, I really grew up. I learned to analyze everything I did. I learned to pull myself apart and stick the pieces back together. I explored Darwin's Theory of Evolution along with the workings of the human brain. I studied several theories that taught different ways to think and to counsel. Everything I learned was interesting and seemed to be valuable, but nothing seemed to really solve anyone's problems. Those I counseled were better for a period of time, but usually they came back in a worse state than before. I began to doubt my skills as a counselor.

Finding a New Body

It was only then that my Spirit Guides intervened. They gently introduced me to a new way of thinking and seeing. I learned that the energy of the human body had to go somewhere besides off into space: it went inwards. My explorations led me to discover the *Etheric Body*. My Spirit Guides taught me how the Etheric Body stored all our emotional and mental experiences from this life in the form of energy. I watched people, fascinated by the way this part of their auras constantly altered. I learned how everyone's Etheric Body has an energy field of its own which flows in a clockwise direction up and back down the body. I noted how, in many people, the more negative their experiences, the more swollen and compacted this body became. Often, I saw the Etheric Body overloaded with wasted energy, which sat dormant, causing a block in its natural flow. I saw how these blocks eventually caused disease and death.

I wanted to explain this to everyone, but whenever I tried, I found my clients too locked into the way they thought and felt. They were threatened by my ideas and began to stay away, so I stopped talking about this and waited. My Spirit Guides continued to teach me how the Etheric Body was a valuable tool through which the Spirit Body learned about the Earth and its ways.

The Right Time and Place

After three years of marriage and the arrival of two sons, I was free again to go on with my life as a healer. I was twenty-three and ready for a new way of life.

Partial massage had become the 'in' thing in England. Having been a nurse, I was well trained in this art. My Spirit Guides wasted no time in teaching me how to make my own aromatherapy oils. As soon as I had successfully made a bottle of lavender or rose oil, there would be a knock on my door or the telephone would ring. It was always someone requesting that I treat a part of his or her body. I practiced on injured arms, legs, feet and backs. I massaged them with my oils, while placing my treasured crystals on their body. During those years, I watched energy flow as I knitted bones, sealed torn ligaments and did what was supposedly the impossible — cure people of their ailments.

During all that time, my Spirit Guides supported me and encouraged me in everything I did. They always gave me a running commentary on what I was doing. Sometimes they directed my treatment of individuals, while other times they left me to use my inspiration.

My children found lost stray cats and dogs that needed healing. Even my own animals brought me mice and birds to heal! Word got out around the neighborhood that I was a healer and they too brought me their sick animal friends. It was a magical time for me. Whenever I worked on an animal, my Spirit Guides were there to direct me. I learned so much about the animal kingdom and how similar they are to humans. In fact, their auras and the way they store or use energy in their Etheric Bodies was no different. Little by little, I learned more about the energy flow of the Physical Body and how it connected to the Etheric Body.

As time passed, my Spirit Guides patiently taught me how the Physical Body was not only connected to the Etheric Body, but also to three other bodies. I learned of the existence of energy patterns that flowed from the

Spirit Body, along with energy from two more bodies, the Higher Mind Body, and the Soul Body. All these bodies entwined in a swirling mass of color, which I easily recognized, from my childhood, as the Aura.

Seek and Ye Shall Find

I became fully established as a Medium, Healer and Counselor with the Spiritualist Association of Great Britain by the time I was twenty-five. That year, I married again and by the time I was thirty, had two more wonderful sons. My life became busy with family affairs, but somehow I managed to continue my spiritual work. I practiced my ministry by serving as a guest medium in various churches in and around London and Essex. My sermons were always given in trance in those days and people came from far and wide to hear what Spirit had to say through me. The Churches were always full and my two oldest sons often accompanied me. It pleased me because I finally had two individuals who didn't question my 'gift' but rather wanted to learn from me. All four of my children were, like me, natural healers and very psychic.

In their own way, each one tested me and brought me to greater awareness about the Etheric Body and the junk that we hold on to through excuses, rationalizations, judgments, guilt, etc. Through observation of my children, I watched their Spirit Bodies develop in the physical sense and came to understand the power of the Spirit Body and its effect on the Etheric and Physical everyday self. Whenever they were sick, I practiced on them.

My Spirit Guides taught me how to see their lessons, and how to help each child know himself and his full potential. I saw myself in them. I saw all the members of my family in them. I saw my family's history in them. I watched as they each molded themselves into their own identities. They were so alike and yet so different. Through general observation of others, I learned about the power of will and the harm it can cause when used negatively. My Spirit Guides showed me how important it was that the Physical, Etheric and Bodies remain in alignment.

Knock And It Will Be Opened Unto You

I put my theories into practice on my clients. I tested My Spirit Guides. I learned very quickly about the power of these three bodies when aligned.

Miracles could occur. However, why some, and not others? Often I had desperately tried to heal some dear sweet soul and failed, while another who seemed unworthy received a cure. I often spent hours telling individuals how to change for the better, only to find them clinging to old ways. Why was it that no one heeded the wisdom I had to share?

My Spirit Guides have a way of answering my questions with events that occur out of the blue. My investigation was halted as I became burdened with another failing marriage.

As often as I could, I tried to heal myself without much success. To cap it all, I was diagnosed as having Parkinson's Disease, inherited from my grandmother. How could I, a healer, knowing so much, be ill? I was devastated. I was angry with my Spirit Guides. Why hadn't they prevented this? Didn't I deserve a cure?

Wallowing in my self-pity for weeks, I finally had a breakdown. The tranquilizers I had been taking were too much for my body and I died. I remember everything about that night. I pleaded with my Spirit Guides to let me stay with them. Their disappointment was never stated, but I felt it. I knew I was letting the team down. I knew I had to go back and try again. They urged me to 'live' and promised me that things would be different. My revival amounted to a new look at 'me' and the knowledge that I had acquired. The door to a new consciousness had been opened, but I didn't know it then.

I questioned, "Where did my knowledge come from?" "Was it my brain or something else?" I had knocked and the door had opened within me.

Ask And Ye Shall Receive

During my recovery, I decided that I didn't want to suffer with Parkinson's Disease and was determined to cure myself. To do it, I had to surrender to my Spirit Guides. My journey inward took me into a whirlpool of my mind. So much of it was false, learned experiences that clouded my vision. I had to find the truth and the truth was somewhere inside.

Over the next five years, I worked diligently with my Spirit Guides who helped me explore with my crystals. By then, I had a large collection of angular stones, which had points protruding. Once I understood the basic technique, I learned more by experimentation and observation on myself. I found I could stimulate, retard, harmonize, tone and balance my energies. My Spirit Guides would stand by and watch me. Whenever I asked a question, they simply told me the answer. During those years, communication with them became extremely easy. My Psychic senses were acute.

In the past, Chakras had just been places on which to put energy into my clients to build up their auras. Now I studied my Chakras, vortices of energy, and learned how they were made and how they worked. I awakened daily to the energy of my Spirit Body and it's power. I healed myself!

I began to have innate knowledge surface across the pictures of my conscious mind. I wasn't an old soul — I was ancient! "Really!" I thought. "So what! What next?"

Revelation Leads to Revolution

'What next' was a revelation! My mind was a dustbin full of rubbish — learned habits, beliefs, disciplines, restrictions and self-inflicted limitations alongside a bowl filled with mixed emotions. All of these served only to keep me depressed, repressed and suppressed — away from the truth. What was the truth? I had a choice. I could change. I decided to change the way I thought and with it the way I saw things in the world. I was still shaking, but at least I had a better attitude, or so I thought! Actually, I was fooling myself. I had simplistically revealed the problem, but changed nothing. I masked everything under a new heading: *Awareness.*

What I needed was a revolution and Spirit gave it to me. They took me on a journey to my ancient past. I saw some of my old lives. I was shocked and stunned, but relieved. My healing skills were mine by right. I hadn't earned it. It wasn't a 'gift' from God. It was a way of life. Pure thought! Pure unconditional Love! This flowed through my Higher Mind Body. My insight was total recall. I knew then that I had to change my brain patterns. I had to change my neural pathways.

Choosing The Right Path And Staying On It

My Spirit Guides told me that there are 144 neural pathways through the brain. I cannot prove this, but do know that when I was ready to change my neural pathways, I had to prepare myself with Crystal Acupuncture^sm. All my Five Bodies had to be flowing and all my Chakras had to be fully rotating at maximum vibration. For several weeks, I worked on myself. I constantly noticed old mindsets that tried to block any changes that may arise. I was facing self-made fears. Little by little, I let go of my thought patterns. I spent much of my time in meditation.

So, on a special night, when all was quiet and my boys were away, I lay down with my Spirit Guides beside me. With their help, I watched energy from a single thought follow along a familiar route around my body, and end up at my fingertips and toes. I learned how each thought followed a familiar pathway. Again and again, I watched old thoughts of fear, pain, and anger and guilt flow around my body, and each time I saw the physical results.

All my nerves were overactive and I shook and trembled badly. My Spirit Guides showed me how to redirect my thoughts along a new neural pathway. I had to feel the emotions of fear, and consciously send that feeling to my brain through a different pathway. They helped me to visualize the journey back to the brain. I watched energy flow like a current of electricity up towards my brain. There I allowed myself to visualize and create a new neural pathway. I made a choice to accept this new pathway. In this way, I spent hours redirecting my energy to flow through the brain, burning new neural pathways stimulated by my emotions. I made one for love to replace anger; one for pleasure to replace fear; one for positive action to replace pain, one for union to replace guilt and one for spiritual growth and independence to replace co-dependency. I knew that in the days, weeks and years to come, I would build new awareness that would become pleasant memories, allowing the old memories to fade and die. In this state of awareness, I knew that my Parkinson's Disease was a manifestation of all the negative traits I had ever accepted within myself.

The next morning, my shakes had practically disappeared. Over the weeks to come, when old fears arose, I began to shake again. This was a reminder to deal purposefully with my attitude and to calmly sort out my emotions by dealing with my problems differently. I was consciously learning to re-program myself. I was a child learning about life and self all over again.

Being An Example Can Be Fun

Once more, I had to make a choice to get divorced and move on with my life. Little by little, everyday events fell into place and I began to rebuild my career. I opened Sumaris Psychic Education Centre and began to treat individuals with all the knowledge that I had acquired in helping myself to overcome Parkinson's disease. My Spirit Guides brought me clients who were more than grateful to subject themselves to me. They did everything I asked without question and the results were astounding. I saw many a transformation in personality and attitude.

The more I worked, the more I was asked to lecture on my successes. I found great pleasure in being with people, unlike my past, where I had struggled to exist in a world of chaos. I remarried and moved to America, where I re-established Sumaris Psychic Education Center, under my Charter as a minister of The Universal Christ Church. As a minister, I was able to function within the law. My work continued as I evolved my healing techniques. I watched individuals develop a whole new persona and a life with meaning, where before there had only been despair. I watched their bodies rejuvenate. Everyone looked younger. I myself, at forty-five, looked younger than I did at thirty-five.

As the years went by, I traveled about the world teaching and healing. All the time I was perfecting my knowledge and techniques. Those who wished to be trained by me took my courses and are now established therapists themselves. Now, at this stage in my life, I have sufficient knowledge to pass on to you, the reader, in the hope that you too can help yourself and those you encounter.

CHAPTER 2

Things My Spirit Guides Taught Me …
And Other Things I Learned By Myself

You Have Five Bodies To Look After

In my Crystal Acupuncture[sm] booklet and at the back of this book, several drawings reveal the natural flow of the Five Bodies that make up the whole you. Those bodies, as mentioned earlier, are the Physical, Etheric, Spirit, Higher Mind and Soul. Each body has its own direction and rate of flow of energy. Each, however, can be affected by another body's energy flow, rather like the waters of two rivers meeting where they become choppy and disturbed. In a normal, healthy Physical Body, the other four bodies flow evenly and rhythmically through the physical form. Unhealthy bodies become swirling masses of energy that often cause riptides within the flow, ultimately developing into physical disease.

The flow of the Five Bodies is controlled by the Main Chakras, *(see diagrams at the back of this book)* vortices of energy, which are in themselves whirlpools of energy. The rotation of each vortex creates a natural resistance to unwanted negative energy. Unfortunately, most people on this planet are open and receptive to negativity in one form or another. As a result, these chakras weaken and spin at a reduced speed that allows outside energy to be drawn into the Physical Body and then on into the Etheric Body and possibly even into the Spirit Body. Excess negative energy will cause a breakdown in the flow of energy throughout these bodies. The result is that that individual will become negative, even suicidal.

The Physical and Etheric Bodies are, by spiritual standards, very dense and coarse. Their vibration is, however, ideal in an earthly sense as the human form is made for a three-dimensional world. The Physical Body dies and become dust. The energy of the Etheric Body is likened to electricity. Its energy can be stored or dissipated without concern for itself. When the Physical Body dies, the Etheric Body disappears, eventually having discharged its energy into the Earth.

The Spirit Body, however, is different. Its energy is compacted spiritual energy which is of the cosmos and, therefore, more refined. The Higher Mind and Soul Bodies are even more refined energy particles of the Universal consciousness and the Universal Love that is called God.

There is a saying in the spiritual sense, "As above, so below." Many examples of that can be seen around us. My analogy of the energy of the Physical Body is like hot mud that slowly moves along its course. The Etheric Body is like thunder and lightening that swell and then discharge as it dies, causing changes in the Physical Body.

The Spirit Body is like the rays of the sun. It warms the Physical Body with bright light and gives it life while clearing away the storms of The Etheric Body. The Higher Mind Body is like a gentle breeze that caresses the Spirit Body, giving it motivation and purpose. The Soul Body, like a blue diamond, is so rare that, it can only be glimpsed as a moment of pure joy. That moment of joy gives an exquisite love that simply washes negativity aside in all Five Bodies.

The energies of the Five Bodies are very different from one another, and yet their very difference is the very reason they are bonded to one another. Opposites attract! It is the nature of the universe to follow the Laws of Karma. In this case: Like attracts like, either in opposition or support for growth without judgment. The Spirit Body needs the Physical Body to experience the ways of the Earth and through its life, to connect with the Universal Consciousness. This way it can test itself and learn to trust itself to evolve and become God.

The Etheric Body is a very necessary link for the Spirit Body to keep its attachment to the Physical Body. In the Etheric Body, all memories of the physical life's existence are stored, together with the Spirit's emotional and mental awareness.. The Etheric Body is the battleground for good and bad to fight it out. Within this body, the earthly mind must fuse with the Spirit mind. Consciousness creates feelings that emanate more energy. Emotional stimuli cause the Physical Body to become active. As a human form, the Spirit must learn to accept the limitations of the flesh and to honor and respect the life it has and the things that it can do. It must also learn to honor and love those it encounters, no matter how hard the way.

In the final analogy, your Physical Body is like your car, and the Etheric is the fuel it runs on. Your Spirit Body is the real you, seeking a way to touch the Universal Consciousness through the Higher Mind Body. In a nutshell, your homework for the next eighty years or so is to drive your car around and not run out of fuel while you go to college every day. You will study hard to learn as much as you can, so that you can graduate with honors and feel great about yourself and ultimately feel connected to the Universe. Then you will feel your Soul Body, that is God within you.

You Are Not Who You Think You Are!

Well now, knowing the above makes things sound easier. Or does it? Actually, at this stage in your awareness, it doesn't. Everyone has been conditioned to think the same way others think. In my book "The Rejection Syndrome," I explain how we are taught to be something we are not. We learn to reject ourselves, our talents and skills, even our own beliefs in the hope that we will fit in with everyone else's point of view in order to be loved. Even the few who think themselves the rebel are conditioned to rationalize themselves away with such sayings as "I'm not important, but my work is" or "I'm different from everyone else, so I have to tell them or teach them my way." or "I'll sacrifice my life to help them." Of course, there are many such sayings in each of us. We rationalize, justify, explain, excuse, and even fantasize with illusions to validate our existence, rather than take a long look and see what is really true.

Yes, we fight tooth and nail to keep our points of view; we will even go to war to protect our point of view. Violence of course is not the answer.

Usually, the wounded parties concerned end up destroying the very way of life that they fought to keep. Nothing stays the same. Change is constant. The one thing you can be sure of in life is to expect the unexpected. In the same way, you can expect your Five Bodies to constantly change, but you cannot control how it changes. Hence the saying, "Go with the flow."

Discover What You Are Really Are!

The first question in anyone's mind should be "Who am I?" With research, it will be made clear that you are your mother in all ways, having lived inside her for six months or more. You have shared your spirit with hers and have become her. When born, you took on her character, her thoughts, hope, dreams etc and tried to keep up with her. What a tall order for a small child! How can you possibly know what she wants all the time? You're not inside her any more. Yet you strive to keep on trying and as you do, you copy everything she is. She is your role model, good and bad. Then there are Dad, Grandpa, uncles, aunts and strangers too all asking you to share yourself with them. Dad's character is hard to copy, but you try. Why, you even copy all the others too! By the time, you are an adult; you have become all those people. A complex adult, full of wonderful hopes and dreams of what you are to become, yet scared to death to take a step towards independence. Scared to be different, in case you don't fit in. What then — A life without love, without friends.; An outcast? Horror!

Take A Leap Of Faith And Change!

Face your fears. Be Independent. Cast out those characters and personality traits that you abhor. Keep the good ones and move on. Blend the remaining characters into what is to become a unique you. Yes, be different. Change your ways. You won't be alone for long. Someone who is like you when you have changed will come along. You cannot escape that Fourth Law of Karma, "Like attracts like." Making new friends brings in new awareness about yourself and your life. You may move away from home, take up new work, or immigrate to far off lands. Whatever you do, it will seem as if life has just begun.

Often these changes occur under stress. There are five situations, which are considered the most stressful - a marriage; a birth; a divorce; a death; a move of work or home. All these events take time to arrange and usually need to be done with great care and fortitude. After the event, generally speaking, the participants are exhausted. It is at this time that internal energy flows are at the lowest and it is during this time that changes in emotional and mental attitudes occur. Yes, the Spirit Body connects with the Physical Body and a revelation occurs, causing the Etheric Body to release trapped energy.

Love. Oh, Such Sweet Love! I Could Die For Love!

Often, falling in love is a welcome excuse to change. Important issues quite suddenly seem insignificant. Individuals change their attitude about themselves overnight. Even physical bodily changes occur. Love is a healing experience in itself. Too bad that you expect your partner to keep the magic going to keep you healthy, wealthy and wise. So often, conditional love is mistaken for true love. Conditional love sets up expectations, which in 90% of the time turns out to be a let down. The poor partner doesn't come up to the standards of your expectation. Well, now what are you going to do about that? Change him/her. Make him/her better!

It is hard work trying to get people to change when they don't want to. I know, I tried it! "Look at me, see me, I know what I'm doing. Do as I tell you! You're a fool if you don't." Yes, we have all said that to someone, either aloud or silently. We are so full of opinions. Learned opinions. Which school is the best? Which Church/Temple etc. is the best. Which food is the best? The list goes on and on and you have an opinion about them all. You learned it from someone and took it as your own opinion. Can you think for yourself? Change your mind. Of course, you can.

Here's Looking At You!

When you look in the mirror. What do you see? Do you like what you see or are you busy comparing notes about yourself with everyone else that you have ever seen? Is the pressure on? Do you want to be slimmer, fatter, smaller, larger, stronger etc. Well, so does everyone else, and yet no one admits it. Everyone tries to fool himself or herself into believing that they are comfortable being themselves, yet as soon as someone says something or gives that look! Well, we just go all to pieces! Where did the confidence go?

Of course, we cannot have opinions without blocking groups of them together to justify everything. We are very clever at making up boxes for this and that. Our brain is an expert in analysis. A real computer is running inside your head. It is even all cross–referenced, like the time you ate ice cream before lunch and were scolded linked with the time you scolded yourself over your weight issues. You can't forget a thing. Your sub-conscious makes sure of that.

Your conscious mind does not remember everything, so it's easy to fake it and say you do not know. But those dreams in the night! They wake you up with a fright. You remember— Horror! You can't break free of the memory. You have to do something about it. You'll worry, and argue with yourself. You'll toss and turn through the night. You'll exhaust yourself and while away the night, angry at your life.

Friend or Foe!

Now you worry about your life and family. Some of them seem careless, lost in their minds, while others physically sap your energy as they describe every detail of their strife. You want to tell them to leave you alone to get on with the changes, but as soon as you try, they emotionally blackmail you to stay the same. They haunt you with their problems and blame you for their mistakes, and you fight for survival, by justifying your relationship with them. You remember the effort you've spent in the past, and the love acts you given, all hopeless, alas. You can't give them up. You might be alone, lost in a sea of hopelessness. Wouldn't that be better than all that pain?

> Some people are flamboyant, while others are shy.
> Some are overpowering, while others are plain boring.
> Still others are dominant freaks of control
> while those that are lazy are distant and droll.
> Where are the few who are gentle, loving and warm?
> Why are they gone when you're mad, ugly and worn.
> Yes, to find the best, you must be the best.

Soul searching is a pathway that we must all take and it only comes into the conscious mind when you cease to compare and begin to accept that you are both the same as and different from everyone else. In the Oneness of the Universal Consciousness all is accepted and all is pleasing, even the dark side. Yes, the dark side highlights the light side. Without both, there can be no appreciation. It is the same within you. You must accept the good and bad within and learn to enjoy who you are.

I Remember When

Once you have decided upon a course of change, you must find the emotional stimuli that will inspire you to make a start. Emotions are the glue that makes things stick to you. You easily remember all the bad things that happened to you because of the traumatic feelings that accompanied the event. Unfortunately, the happy events seemed to slip away. We haven't been trained to remember those. I remember my mother saying things like, "That ... was so bad, I'll remember that for as long as I live." I also remember such statements as "I wish I were dead." "I'll never forgive you." "I hate myself."

I can quite honestly say that I never heard anyone say, "This was the best day of my life, and I'll remember it as long as I live." I said it to myself the day I delivered my first child and on that day, I made a promise to look for those wonderful moments in the future. As the years went by however, I still noticed the bad days. It took me another fifteen years to really see the good in each day of my life.

You Are Ruled By God's Laws Of Karma!

Every day is a special day. It is a chance to take another look around you and try something new, or do something differently. It is a day to meet new people, learn about new things and grow. It is one more day to enjoy being you and to taste the goodness that God has created. But, how can that be, you may well ask? With guns and robbers, murderers and villains on the prowl full of drugs, alcohol and tobacco, how can I feel safe? That Fourth Law of Karma "Like attracts like," must rear its head again. If you fear it, you attract it. Don't notice it, and it will pass you by. The first Law of Karma is "No fragment (individual) may impose its will on another at anytime on any level". If you don't look for trouble, you are not inviting it, so it has to leave you alone. If you dream of danger, you are attracting it. So, clean up your fears.

There are five Laws of Karma in all *(see back of this book)*. These are fully explained in my book, *The Way to Oneness*. However, for those who are reading about them for the first time, here is number three. "Each fragment shall share itself with all other fragments in unconditional love."

Yes, under this law you must give the time of day to those in need, should they seek you out. Bear in mind that if they do, you too need help. This Fourth Law of Karma as mentioned frequently above is "Each fragment shall attract like in the mirror image, either in opposition or support for growth without judgment."

The Second Law of Karma is "Each fragment shall be responsible for all it creates in positive and negative actions." This literally means that if you broke it you fix it, which of course includes yourself. Don't expect others to make you feel better. Be responsible for your own choice of feelings. A broken heart is a state of mind, and the emotion that makes it an issue is greed. "I want him. I can't live without him." You can change your mind in a blink of the eye.

The Fifth Law of Karma is "Each fragment shall, in unconditional love, surrender to the Creator." In a nutshell, this means that your will must be the will of God. If you want to get ahead, you must read the signs. God gives signs. The trouble is most of us don't see them. Here's a tip. Look behind the event that seems to block you. What are you learning? What haven't you seen about yourself and your situation yet? When you find an answer do not conclude that that is all. Look deeper. Sometimes the answer is hidden behind shallow answers. Remember the ultimate answer is to do with spiritual growth and the love of God.

Take time out now and have a think about your life to date. Has it been a happy road or was it full of potholes? Did you make those potholes or did you fall into someone else's. Are you ready to begin afresh? Then let's proceed.

CHAPTER 3

Physical And Emotional Issues

You Look Like You Feel.

So far, you have read a lot about conditioning and not much about of Crystal Acupuncture^{sm} & Teragram^{sm} Therapy. Be patient and I will get you there eventually. Let us first look at what are called Body Syndromes. These are areas of the Physical Body where energy from the Etheric Body can be blocked, preventing Spiritual Body energy from connecting and flowing into the Physical Body.

Is The Responsibility Too Much? (The 3 Primal R's)

If you have been trying to "control" people and/or deal with issues in your life, then you will be carrying the three causes *Resistance, Resentment and Rejection*. You will have been breaking the First Law of Karma, by imposing your will on someone else. You will be steeped in the Responsibility Syndrome, which affects the head, neck, shoulders and upper back. Your Aura will be dominantly red and you will be very angry. Yes your shoulders will feel as though they are about to snap. Headaches and neck cramps will plague you. Various illnesses in these areas will occur if the situation you are living in is unresolved.

Who Cares About Me Anyway? (The 3 Transition R's)

If you have been seeking sympathy and support, telling about yourself, while feeling weak and incapable of dealing with situations in your life, then you are caught up in the Crying Syndrome. You are not applying the Second Law of Karma to yourself. You must take responsibility for all your actions, whether good or bad, take a chance, and change your life for the better. Often the causes for being stuck in this syndrome are an awareness of a *Revelation*, and a need to have a *Revolution* to bring about a *Resolution*.

The longer you resist responsibility for your change the more your face; throat, chest, heart and solar plexus will be effected. Your Aura will be predominantly yellow as you argue back and forth around the changes.

Get into your heart and follow your feelings. Trust yourself and change for the better.

It's Impossible To Be Successful If…(The 3 focal P's)

If you are in a relationship problem, whether intimate, business, family or social which does not seem to clear, then you are caught in the Sexual/ Guilt Syndrome. Somehow, you are breaking the third Law of Karma. You are not sharing yourself with those who are at loggerheads with you. You have not found out how to love them in spite of the situation. Something in you is trying to change something that should be left as it is. Look at your *perception*. Are you too *Persistent*? Maybe you are too dominant. Where is your *power*? Is it down the tubes? Did you tell a truth or a lie to try and manipulate the situation? If you did, then get out of it right now. Your Aura is green. Who do you envy? Unconditional love says walk away and come back another day when you've got your head on straight and your heart in the right place.

I Don't Know How Or Why (The 3 Harmonic A's)

Are you in a lover's abyss, lost in "what was?" Hoping to renew it "as it was"? If so, then you are preventing changes from occurring. Perhaps you are stuck in a rut, wanting changes to occur, but are too afraid to make them. Then you are caught in the Flight Syndrome. Take a look at yourself. There you are clinging with those fingers to the ledge. Afraid to fall! Your lower arms and armpits are twisted in agony as you hold on. You mid-back is about to break. Your tummy is churning endlessly and your feet ache, especially the toes as you tip toe along the edge.

Your Aura is deep blue. You are depressed. Are you so afraid to make a change? Your mind has got you in turmoil. You do not know if you are coming or going. You must come to an *agreement* with yourself, to make an *acceptance* that the past is done. Give yourself *absolution* and let go. Fall and trust yourself that you will survive. Remember the Fourth Law of Karma. You will meet others like you and in the mirror- image; you will grow to love them without judgment.

No One's Interested In Me, So... (The 3 Eternal "E's)

So you don't believe you can have better? You think things are safe if you hide in a rut? Wrong! You have forgotten about your needs. You need to have an *existence* full of *experience* that will allow your Spirit to take its natural course in *evolution* towards God. Remember the Fifth Law of Karma. You must love unconditionally and surrender to the Creator. In turn you must surrender to yourself and develop creative pursuits that will expand your awareness. If you don't, your hips, legs knees and feet along with your hands, elbow and back will give you trouble. Why? Because you're in the fighting position, desperately making a last stand to survive with old habits. Throw them away. Turn your dark purple Aura into lavender and be happy. Grow spiritually. Get a life!

Walk With Your Head Held High!

Whatever your Body Syndrome, and you may be suffering with more than one, your muscles and bones will be affected as you hold your body in rigid postures. Nerve endings will hurt as you strain and knot the muscles. Bones will crack and ligaments will snap. You will be out of alignment and need to see a chiropractor. He'll straighten you and for awhile you'll feel better as energy begins to flow again, but as soon as you get back into your old routine, that Body Syndrome will pop right back in. So, whatever your situation, you will need to lose the past and make major changes in your attitude to life and move through the "Stages of Loss".

You Can Have More!

Anger is the first Stage of Loss. It is human nature to be in denial of approaching changes. Whether you argue with yourself or others, there will come a time when you will see all your arguments as useless. When this occurs, you will grow angry with those around you. You will *blame* and *shame* them for your circumstances. In time, you will turn that anger inward as you realize in *sorrow* that only you are responsible for your state of well being.

Once you focus on your negative emotions, you will become *miserable* and wallow in *depression* and *failure* as you enter *abandonment* in the Second Stage of Loss. You will mourn the loss of what was for a while. Eventually, you will overcome depression, as you begin to bargain with yourself.

Bargaining is the Third Stage of Loss. This allows you to set up scenarios for a new life pattern. In time, your bargaining ideas will seem attractive and you will stimulate yourself to seek a resolution to your situation. At that point, you will embrace the Fourth Stage of Loss, providing *acceptance* of *closure* on the past as a new door opens into your happy future.

You Are A Living, Walking Record Of Your Own History!

Everything that I have mentioned in the previous pages has happened to you. All your experiences have been stored in the cellular-neuro-muscular memory of your body. In other words, every cell has your intimate life encoded into it. Every physical movement you have made is trapped in the memory and cross-referenced into every emotional experience. It is then filed into sections under headings that group your experiences together, either collectively, or separately. These memories are both good and bad and are stored in the form of pictures. If I ask you to think of a tank, you will see a tank or part of it. If I ask you to make association with that tank, you will pull up other pictures. Each picture you see provides you with a wealth of information from your past.

As you recall these experiences, your body reruns the tension that was felt in the muscles at that time. If it was a bad time in your life, the metabolic rate of your body will change and you will become anxious, although your present situation is calm. You will rationalize that you are having a panic attack. I will go one step further and say that you are doing it all over again.

You Can Be Healthy And Free!

Deprogramming the cellular-neuro-muscular memory is a must. Crystal Acupuncture^sm and Teragram^sm Therapy are excellent tools to make these changes. However, I emphasize that counseling sessions are also necessary. As each cell in the body is changed, chemical, biochemical, emotional and mental changes will occur that eventually allow a spiritual change to occur.

Each cell has emanations of the Five Bodies running through it. By changing the rate of flow in one body, it will affect the flow of the other four bodies in that cell. Since cells are tiny and very close together, it is impossible to physically demonstrate the changes, especially since the Spirit Body, Higher Mind Body and Soul Body are hard to see unless you are psychic.

Unfortunately, no scientist would believe a psychic! I had to wait twenty years for professors at the London University to validate my statement that the neural spine will heal if the broken ends are placed together. Then those with broken backs would walk again. I was twenty then and very hurt when they laughed at me. By the time they would prove me right, I had already helped spines to mend. My problem was getting the patients to accept full recovery. A break in C4 meant a life spent lying down. My patients settled for a life with full use of the arms and body. Why didn't they walk? In their minds, they didn't deserve a miracle. I was up against beliefs.

Trust With The Heart Of A Child And Believe In The Magic!

Beliefs are learned experiences that have been accepted while in a hypnotic state. When visual observation and emotional expression validate these beliefs, then the belief becomes obsession. An example, would be the antiquated belief that God is only in Humans, not in animals. How could one know the truth? As a child we listen and accept all that is shown to us with wide eyes. We carry many of those beliefs throughout our lives. Sometimes those beliefs block us from growing. Perhaps it is time for you to look at your beliefs. I know that I had to discard many of my childhood beliefs, especially the ones I concocted myself, such as, "I never get to be first."

As I shed one belief after another, I always found a new belief. Eventually some of those beliefs changed too. Beliefs are only good as long as they help you to grow. Beliefs that hold you down create fear, pain, anger and guilt as well as loneliness. The greatest hurt of all is to feel unloved. Do you love yourself, or do you believe yourself unworthy of love? Take a test. Buy yourself something nice and see if you feel good about receiving it!

Negative emotions prevent your spirit from growing. If your mind is loaded with fear, pain, anger and guilt, then your emotions will force your body into deformity. Illness is inevitable. If you have done wrong, then you must forgive yourself and draw comfort from the experience, knowing that you are now wiser for having made the mistake and a better person for having had the bad experience. From a spiritual point of view, nothing is truly bad. Everything is simply an experience that we move through to be awakened to a desire to be closer to God.

You Can Save Yourself With Crystals!

Those who suffer seek God in their lives. They ask to be saved. Remember that God knows that no one needs to be saved. They only need to see the way to help themselves. There is always someone to help when you call out.

As a Therapist, I help many clients in times of need. Of course, I know that I can only help those who truly want to be helped. Many cry out, but few are really ready to change. For some, it is too scary to change. They just want a hug, and then go merrily on their way, until the charge runs out. Then they come back for another hug. Eventually, anger will cause a desire to end running from change. When Crystal Acupuncture[sm] Therapy is applied, each cell is very subtly changed as the crystals amplify, tone and balance the energy flow of the Five Bodies at the cellular level, as well as through each of the Five Bodies.

To try to understand a simple cell with energy flowing through it, let's first think of a circle. Now in your mind, draw a black line across it. This represents the energy of the Physical Body. Now draw a red line directly perpendicular to the black line forming a cross in the circle. This red line is the Etheric Body's energy. Now take a yellow line and draw an inner circle, close to the edge of the cell, This is the Spirit Body 's energy. It crosses over the Physical and Etheric Bodies. Now take a blue line and cross the cell on the diagonal to the cross made by the Physical and Etheric Bodies. This is the Higher Mind Body.

Now take a green line and cross over the other diagonal. This is the pathway of the Soul Body. The interaction of energy in each cell keeps it alive and rejuvenated. When a cell breaks down and grows abnormally, it is diseased. This represents an imbalance in the flow of energies. One small block in one small cell can lead to mass deterioration of many cells. That original block could quite simply be a lack of self-appreciation in relation to a memory involving that part of the body, where early childhood damage took place. It could be just a simple graze that in later years leads to cancer.

Crystal Acupuncture can force those early memories to the surface. By stimulating the cellular-neuro-muscular memory in that area, pictures from the past bring old negative emotions into the conscious mind. By counseling in open dialogue, ideas can be changed. Emotions can be healed. Energies can then flow again, allowing physical healing to occur.

CHAPTER 4

The Ravages Of Conditioning

I Can't Understand, But I Can Smell The Difference!

You could say, "I can smell a rat." I have talked a lot about conditioning, but what about the more subtle things that just seem to happen to us? For example, those allergies that just seem to grab us and pull us down for no apparent reason, or those little intuitive moments, when something doesn't feel right! Everyone has a keen sense of smell and/or taste along with inner feelings. Our acceptance or rejection of flavor and smell is a very individual choice. Although a mother may inform her child that onions are wonderful to eat, it does not necessarily follow that the child will like them too.

If we are given the chance to try things for ourselves, then we make up our own minds about them. Unfortunately, many parents inform their children that certain foods are not nice and should be avoided at all cost. Mother doesn't like it, so she doesn't buy it. The child then adopts her policy and is conditioned to accept the idea that that particular food is horrible. It is not unusual for adults to rediscover food and claim a new favorite.

You Are What You Eat!

If life were always pleasant and meals were always divine, then everyone would have a healthy appetite. Unfortunately, meal times are often the only time when families get together, and if there is anger in the house, it is most likely to rear its head around the dinner table. Babies and children under eight years old will absorb more than food. As they eat, with the use of Psychometry, they feel their parents and older siblings. Whatever emotions are thrown around the table are stored in association with the food the child is eating. Years later, a quite healthy meal can be a physical stimulus to press the emotional button and bring up childhood fears, pain, anger, guilt and hurt. This can also work in reverse. Foods associated with comforting times can be yearned for in times of stress.

Familiar Places And Faces Have Smells Too!

Of course, the world is full of different smells beyond the kitchen. The brain stores memories of pictured events along with aromas of varying kinds. Putrid smells are not necessarily remembered as bad smells if the event at the time was handled well emotionally. Sweet smells, such as flowers and honey, could cause alarm if a child has a bee sting associated with it, or an over-bearing aunt who wore perfume. Panic attacks are often caused by subconscious outbreaks of fear from an association of smells or tastes.

Remember that, although your conscious mind cannot recall the memory, your sub-conscious mind can. Even the words are all there. The only way to find out about your reaction is to go into a state of meditation or hypnosis to find out and maybe that is not such a good idea! Some fears, though very childish, are best left alone. They can be overcome with mind control suggestions. In hypnosis, we use a double bind. For example, "The more you feel afraid of spiders, the more you like them." It works! These two commands are direct contradictions and the mind only knows one way to deal with opposing commands. That is to be neutral. Spiders don't matter any more.

If you have strange allergies, phobias, nightmares and panic attacks, then you are making associations with the past. Your Etheric Body needs cleansing. Your Lower Earthly Mind is out of control. You have an imbalance in the way you see, touch and feel things. Your mind is in illusions and fantasies. When Crystal Acupuncture^{sm} is used in these circumstances, these problems will surface. It is important to use Teragram^{sm} Therapy as well, along with Hypnotherapy.

Dispel The Monster In The Closet And Be A Hero!

All fears, whether real or false, are encoded in every cell. When you decide to face your fears, you must be prepared to deal with the monster inside you. That monster is your conscious mind. It lies to you and cheats on you. It fools you with stupid ideas that compound your problem. If it is a real fear, it should be discussed with a counselor, while a phobia should simply be pulled apart and destroyed. Both kinds of fear must be eliminated from the body, and replaced with new programming that includes power, strength and confidence. I have found that Hypnotherapy is the best tool to use for my clients. Discussing, analyzing etc. only serves to make the fear worse. Hypnosis allows a person to deal with their fear in a controlled way that gets rid of it immediately. When this kind of treatment is called for, I always use my Teragram^{sm} Therapy. The release of any form of anxiety will call for a re-balancing and rebuilding of the Chakras.

Fear is your friend, not your enemy. It tells you there is something wrong in your perception, which needs to be fixed. If fear is not released, then nervous disorders will manifest, which may end up in the form of a serious complaint such as Parkinson's Disease. When I manifested it, I was full of fear. Once I eliminated my fear, my nerves healed.

Emotional distress will cause major organs to deteriorate. When seeking help, it is important to accept that your mindsets on a conscious level are causing you to suffer emotionally. Whatever rationale you have about your life has to change. If you need to, you must change your way of life.

Once deterioration of the organs occurs, it will take a great many sessions with Teragram^{sm} Therapy and other Therapies such as Reflexology with Aromatherapy, or Shiatsu with deep breathing to open up the meridians so that energy can flow productively. Unfortunately, those who wait too long and find themselves seriously ill are so steeped in negativity, with conditioned resistance to any radical changes, that they prevent healing from occurring. To get better, you have to want it. You have to be hungry for it! So each time you eat something, smell something or simply drink something, stop! Ask yourself a simple question. Do I have any bad memories around this kind of thing? If you do, ask yourself why you are still reacting. The same can be said of something you are looking at. If you have a reaction, stop and ask yourself why. It may be an irrational answer. Look behind that answer. Look for the truth. Then get therapy.

You Are Your Own Reality!

Everything your five senses experienced in the first eight years of your life created your primary mindsets, which travel along the neural pathways of the brain. If you saw it, heard it, felt it, smelt it, tasted it, then you had an emotional response. Your childish mind tried to make sense of that experience. Nine times out of ten, it was the wrong assessment.

Over the years, as you have matured, you have compounded those beliefs with rational thinking that has suppressed those childish fears. Now, as an adult, it is possible for you to make sense of non-sensible garbage stored in your sub-conscious. The way to do this is to tap into your deep subconscious, otherwise known as your Spirit Mind, and find the truth. Crystal Acupuncture[sm] and Teragram[sm] Therapy will help you get there.

Take time to stop and appreciate your eyes and ears. As an infant, you focused on a world full of strange shapes and noises. Every shape had to be recognized and learned. Every noise had a meaning too — a million shapes with a million sounds. Day after day your brain tries to make sense of what is seen and heard, and the only way it can do that is to listen to your feelings. A dog barking and a sudden fright send an emotion of alarm to the brain, which helps you remember the creature. A bee buzzing near your nose, and then out of sight, could give an emotion of anxiety. Of course, these could have been positive experiences. No one can say why you chose to react the way you did. Only you can sift through and find the truth. After all, it is your mind!

Taste, Like Love, Is Better The Second Time Around!

On a conscious level, touch is probably the most dominant of the five senses. A baby touches everything. Everything goes into the mouth. The tongue is one of the most sensitive parts of the body. Everything around a child, be it inanimate or animate, has a vibration. The mouth is extremely sensitive to vibration. In the early years of childhood, Psychometry is constantly used to sense the use and form of what is felt. What better place to assimilate information than the mouth!

Later, as things and people take on names and character, the child learns to speak. Now form has a spoken vibration. Words have resonated in and around the child's Aura. These words may be fierce or loving. The child will react emotionally, causing more stored memories formed around childish associations. Words are a series of tones, which in turn, are quite simply musical notes. Notes vibrate, causing energy to move. Sudden harsh words cause baby's Aura to shift as the energies of the Five Bodies move. This causes a disturbance to the child, which takes him into a new experience. If the experience is not a loving nurturing one, the child will make a negative association, even though the words may not be understood at that time.

To deprogram yourself on such a deep level calls for a total surrender of your way of life. I know this is very scary for most, but when it occurs, there is a great spiritual awakening that allows a total shift in consciousness, followed by a shift in energy and a subsequent new growth of healthy tissue. You can taste again! Sudden confrontations with death can stimulate such a change in awareness.

Let Go, And Let Happen!

Spiritual Crystal Acupuncture℠ helps individuals to move into deep states of meditation in order to follow a quest of discovery. Teragram℠ Therapy helps balance the Chakras during the inner journey. You might say that you get your miracle!

Erasing personal history is a must if you are seriously ill. Your illness is a loud sign that the way you think and feel is wrong for you. By letting go of your conscious mindsets, and then unveiling your subconscious memories, you will reach the truth that lies in your deep-subconscious (Spirit) mind.

CHAPTER 5

Intellectual And Physical
Behavioral Models

I Think, Therefore I Feel. I Feel, Therefore I Think. I Think.
Confusion!

There are two kinds of people in the world. They are Emotional Intellectuals and Emotional Physicals. Emotional Intellectuals do not consider themselves very emotional. Of course, they have as many feelings as anyone else does. Usually they suppress any outbursts by taking any feelings that they are having into the mind, where they seek a logical answer for the feeling. Here the Conscious Mind analyzes everything, causing that individual to become totally lost in thought. They are unaware of what is happening to their body. Slowly over time, they become tense and stressed as they guard themselves against invasion of any kind, especially by the Physical type. Fortunately for them, they are attracted to their opposite, the Emotional Physical type.

Each of us must, under the influence of the Fourth Law of Karma, seek union through our differences in order to learn to erase our opinions of ourselves and anyone else we would judge. If you are an Emotional Intellectual type, you will often live through each day totally unaware of minor symptoms that warn of an impending breakdown in your body.

Unfortunately, many people have a sudden stroke or major malfunction of some part of their body which forces them to take a long look at their way of life and to touch deep-seated emotions that have long been suppressed. Hopefully, if this occurs, they will have a revelation and change the way they are. Sadly, most do not. They rationalize that they are too old to change and play it safe by staying the same. Of course, deterioration sets in. They may bitterly complain about their condition and revel in old memories of how fit they used to be. If this type of person should make a change for the better, then they usually become dedicated to finding new ways to explore themselves, analyzing every move, checking things out to make sure they feel safe. Caution is their friend. If you think you are an Emotional Intellectual, make sure you learn to watch your body for telltale signs that show when you are neglecting your body and your true emotions.

The Emotional Physical types are quite different. They spend most of their lives interested in their body and what it is feeling. They notice every little twitch. They worry about their weight and size. They like to be noticed and complimented, unlike their Emotional Intellectual counterparts, who run away and hide. These Emotional Physical types are demonstrators. They like to talk and share themselves. They want to be loved and felt in the hearts of all those they encounter. It hurts their whole body if they are rejected. They love to dress in flamboyant clothes and often make good performers. If someone upsets them, then their life is ruined until they find closure. Their Emotional Intellectual partner will seem to leave loose ends hanging all over the place, which, of course, is sheer torture for the Physical type who wants to know everything.

Listen, Speak And Learn!

Here is a little advice for you Emotional Physical types who are dealing with sensitive Emotional Intellectual types. When you become emotionally attached to him/her, learn to read behind what is said. Every piece of dialogue you give is received that way. You may be literal and mean what you say, but your partner will think otherwise. "Shut the door please," can mean "It's your fault the last electric bill was so high!" When an Emotional Intellectual asks you what you think. Don't tell him what you feel. He can't equate emotions with his thoughts. Just explain your circumstances.

Little by little you will learn to develop your mind and become a little more balanced between what you feel and what you think.

Here is some advice of those dealing with sensitive Emotional Physical types. Check that what you heard really means what you think it means. Check repeatedly until you are sure and then give your response. Say things like, "I thought you said. Does that mean…" If the answer is "No." Then keep on trying until you understand.

If you are an Emotional Intellectual type and your Physical partner is complaining, know that she/he doesn't want you to necessarily fix h/her problem. What she/he really wants is a hug instead. So, let yourself become more physical. Hug and try to feel what is happening to your emotions and your body. Slowly but surely you will find more physicality within you.

When individuals take time out to work with the Crystal Acupuncture^sm and Teragram^sm Therapies, a lot of progress can be made in being able to harmonize the way you think, with the way you feel. Ideally, everyone should be 50/50. Few are! So it is quite in order to aim for 60/40 percent. This allows one aspect of you to be either a little bit more Emotionally Intellectual, or vice versa.

Who's To Blame? What A Shame

When two high Emotional Physicals bond, it can be torture. Both complain and judge. Arguments go back and forth. Competition sets in. Each feels the other does not care about them. They grow embittered with one another, but refuse to leave. They are constantly seeking closure for all the years of sadness etc. They want praise for their suffering. Most important of all, they want to be drenched in love and appreciation.

When two high Emotional Intellectuals get together, they will have a lot in common in certain areas of their thoughts. They will talk for hours. As soon as that topic is drained, they will become bored with one another. It is not unusual to find a married couple, who are both interested in their careers, their friends and activities outside their homes. So guess what. We don't really have a marriage. We have an arrangement, and arrangements can be broken. Usually, these types of marriages don't last.

I'll Love You Forever At This Moment!

So the best partners are opposites. Each is able to tolerate the other and search for answers. Eventually good solid foundation stones can be laid that lead to a good sound marriage or partnership. Of course, no relationship is perfect in the beginning. Like a good wine, it takes time to mature.

Sexual activities can be a problem for some. The Emotional Intellectual will become very physical for brief periods, during which time he/she will give his/her undying love and attention, though his/her love making may be short in duration. The Physical may complain that there is not enough contact. He/she wants to be in contact for hours. Our reproductive organs are controlled by the flow of energy that passes through the Base/Root Chakra. Of course, this area needs to be re-balanced frequently.

My Spirit Guides pointed out to me how often sexual repression or lack of activity can lead to major illnesses. With their help, I could clearly see how sexual activity is nature's way of moving energies around the Physical Body. An orgasm moves energy though the Five Bodies creating an alignment. Unfortunately, they also helped me to see how some individuals use sexual activity as a way to temporarily stop pain and avoid changes by holding on to unlearned lessons that remain embedded in the Base/Root Chakra. In these cases, energy is unable to find a way through the many blocks that exist in other areas of the body. When sex is good, the Heart Chakra dilates and emotions spill out releasing negativity. At that moment there is a sense of unity that overrides any fear of change. Many promises are made, but very few are remembered later.

I'm Sick And Tired Of The Same Thing!

I learned from my Spirit Guides that another way the energies of the Chakras can be put back into alignment is through vomiting. When people are scared, they often wretch and then feel better afterwards. This physical act causes the Solar Plexus Chakra to restart itself and pick up the speed of its rotation. This kind of rebalancing is always caused by emotional distress. Bulimia is another form of balancing the body. Eating has emotional guilt attached to it. Guilt stimulates the need to vomit. After vomiting, a peace descends upon them temporarily, until they have to eat again.

You Are Never Too Old To Sing And Dance!

For as long as I can remember, I loved to sing. When I was very young, whenever I was upset about something, I quite naturally sang my favorite hate songs. Sometimes I even spontaneously made up tunes to fit my own words. Somehow, I always felt better afterwards. Years later, my Spirit Guides taught me how singing stimulates and balances the Throat Chakra. When this Chakra balances, it automatically effects the Heart and Solar Plexus Chakras. I learned that as these three Chakras spin in rhythm, a good sense of well-being emanates and the Five Bodies harmonize. Listening to music can have the same affect, providing the music has a soothing tone to it. I love to meditate to the sound of music and comforting tones.

Some children like to spin on the spot. This is another way of stimulating the chakras to rebalance and the Five Bodies to align. Unfortunately, as adults, we tend to feel foolish doing childish things. Overcome that inhibition and try it. Don't get too dizzy though. You could fall and hurt yourself, so do it where you know you can land safely. Spin in one direction and then reverse the procedure. End with a clockwise spin. This technique helps the Etheric Body to let go of negativity. You will feel young again.

When we were young we ran and played without a second thought. Physical exercise was a must then and still is now. Stretching, bending, and running on the spot are all just as good as walking or hiking. So, there are no excuses. Stretching and bending will help the glands in your body to work proficiently. Getting your heart rate up will release endorphins into your blood. You'll feel better, and act younger! Your Aura will be radiant.

You Can Follow Directions!

Over the years, I've found myself constantly watching the way I think and the emotions that have arisen as a result of negative mindsets. I learned to redirect my thoughts by using strong emotional desires, firmly placed into pictures of where I saw myself in the future. Though my pictures may have changed, the results kept coming. My Spirit Guides constantly encouraged me to keep myself active and child-like in everything I did. I expected the best. I did my best. I never let anyone stop me from doing what I wanted to do. I just had to adapt a little here and there, in order to get things going.

You too can adapt. During your exercise, you should reprogram your mind with new emotions attached. Remember that emotions are the glue that makes your thoughts stay in your mind. Be as positive as you can and make those ideas as simple as possible. Long sentences lead to excuses and confusion, especially if you are the Emotional Intellectual type. So, take those long sentences and edit them. Here is an example: "I promise myself to get up early every morning and workout, especially on weekends when I don't have to work." Change that to "Workout at 8 am daily plus one extra hour on weekends." The first sentence leaves plenty of room for procrastination. The second sentence is a command. Your brain likes commands. It will accept what you say.

Repetition is not necessary if you add the feeling of joy with the idea. So, picture yourself working out with your favorite music playing while you sing along as you exercise. The next thing you will know is that you are awake by 8 a.m. ready for your workout. Before working out, you can use Crystal Acupuncture^sm. Stimulate your meridians with Quartz and get going. After your workout you can slow yourself down with an Aventurine crystal and take a nice relaxing shower. This way, you will not strain your muscles or suffer the next day.

Silence Is Golden! Hear The Praises!

Take a look at the way you talk to yourself. You may be a chatterbox. If so, try to still your mind by using a discipline such as meditation or hypnosis to correct yourself. Underneath all this chatter are some fears you need to see and erase. Establish new guidelines. Don't criticize yourself. Praise yourself instead.

The way you think about yourself establishes your level of self-esteem. Be positive and build up your self-esteem. Next, be aware of your levels of self-worth. Your talents and skills, along with training are worthy of praise too. You should also effectively use your time productively; making sure your energy is spent well, this way you will build your self-value too. When you feel good about yourself emotionally, mentally and physically, then you will discover inner joy and a love of life.

Meditation Is Powerful And Priceless

Use Crystal Acupuncture^{sm} Therapy to focus on themes that you wish to eliminate from your cellular-neuro-muscular system. Then meditate with Teragram^{sm} Therapy to release this negative energy. Meditate on new positive ideas to replace that which has been changed. Here is an example: I wish to release my need to ask for approval. Use your obelisk cut stone and do Crystal Acupuncture^{sm} *(see diagram at back of this book)* on the main five meridians of both hands. When finished, meditate with the Teragrams on your Chakras *(see diagram at back of this book)*, while lying in a comfortable position. Repeat to yourself several times, "I am releasing my need to receive approval". Watch your body release negative energy. Then repeat your positive statement several times. "I am confident." Your sub-conscious mind will make the necessary changes and in the weeks to come you will notice how you ask less and less for approval.

CHAPTER 6

Images Of The Five Bodies

You Are So Powerful and So Strong and So Beautiful!

Now that you are aware of your mind and emotions and the many different ways you may build energy and block or dissipate it, have you stopped to think about what you really look like? My Spirit Guides showed me what I looked like through my husband, Steve Van Coops. At that time, in the early 1980's, he was using his Mediumship to take Polaroid photos of auric emanations. His pictures were astounding. I would look at a person and see their Aura. Then he would take a photo, and 'Lo and behold', there was the Aura on film along with faces of that person's Spirit Guide. This was a wonderful time in my life, when I finally began to fully realize just how beautiful we all are. Following my Spirit Guides' direction, I went on to specialize in studying the performance and magnificence of the human form.

You Are A Perfect Working Machine

With my own eyes and the eyes of my Spirit Guides, I was able to both see and feel the energies of all my clients who came to me for healing. Through many years of research, I have come to know how powerful and magnificent each of the Five Bodies is. The way they expand and interact, cascading around an individual, is one of the most beautiful things to behold! Unfortunately, most people find it hard to see their emanations or even to feel them. So, perhaps with a little more understanding about how they are formed, their functions, you may open your eyes and see your true self some day.

Each of the Five Bodies has emanations, which collectively form the Aura. In my book, *The Book of Crystal Acupuncture ℠ and Teragram ℠ Therapy Diagrams,* illustrations clearly show the directional flow of the Five Bodies. For your convenience, these have been included at the back of this book. Each cell in the Physical Body has its own life force, which is electro-magnetic. Physical energy is, like the mind, both negative and positive, and as such seeks polarity. Energy is distributed around the body by acts of attracting and repelling. A series of tiny impulses is the result. These impulses stimulate the metabolic rate and subsequent rejuvenation of the cells. Every day, thousands of cells die and an equal number are born.

The Physical Body has a consistent pattern of energy that is similar to a light switching itself on or off. This natural biochemical rhythm creates heat through friction with relative sound waves. Sound waves are a denser vibration than heat waves. Both have a spectrum of colors, which cannot be seen by the naked eye. These colors can vary from dark brown to white depending on the state of the body. A sick person has an Aura full of dark and somber colors, speckled with lighter colors as they try to heal themselves.

A healthy body is full of bright light colors, along with vibrant true colors that show healthy action. Scientists have developed mechanical equipment that can detect these emanations. The Physical Body's energy surges upward toward the brain and then back down again to the feet. This energy flow follows the natural meridians of the body.

The Etheric Body is not so easy to trace. This body is likely to be filled with memories relating to emotional trauma of some kind. As the mind recalls past events, emotional responses stimulate this body to flare outwards. This distribution of energy causes undercurrents in the flow. The more negative a person is, the more turmoil there is in the way the energy flows through this body. Minute whirlpools of energy swirl around in each cell, sometimes causing a disruption of the physical cell. Illness results. Etheric energy, like the Physical energy, flows by impulse.

However, unlike the Physical Body, contraction and expansion cause the flow in this body. Emotional fears, along with pain, anger, guilt, loneliness etc. cause the energy to swell, while memories of happy events cause the energy to reduce. As the sub-conscious mind is constantly shifting through one's history, there are plenty of stimuli to make this body flow rapidly around the Physical Body, causing a physical reaction. The colors of a healthy Etheric Body are white with rainbow swells. An unhealthy Etheric Body is usually a deep green and yellow with splashes of red, white, and occasional dark blue spurts. The emanation of this body can be seen, with a psychic eye, to protrude approximately 2 to 4 inches away from the physical form. Its natural flow is in a spiral clockwise rotation upward towards the brain, then to return to the feet in like manner.

The Spirit Body is not of the Earth. Its make up is of a cosmic nature. Thousands of minute specks create the Spirit Body. These tiny specs of light energy are quite literally attracted to one another. The more there are, the more a form can be seen. The Spirit Body flows like an ocean. It rises and falls to a rhythmic pulse of its own. Because of its expanding nature, a Spirit Body is capable of greatly exceeding the body size. However, in most cases, the Spirit Body is usually around the same size as the human form, with an emanation that can be seen psychically to extend some three feet or more. It always remains in a constant egg shape, the narrow end being at the feet. Each cell in the Physical Body has a collection of tiny Spirit Body specs that manifest in form as ectoplasm, which gives life to it.

As the Physical and Etheric Bodies move by impulse, so that impulse stimulates the Spirit Body to expand and contract. In extreme cases of fear on a conscious level, the Spirit Body will contract, becoming denser and heavier. In this way it can support the body and stimulate new growth. During this time, the Spirit is less aware of its higher consciousness. It is attracted to the Etheric Body, and through that connection, can learn more about itself and its lessons in physical form.

If the Etheric Body is over-burdened with anxiety and fear, the Spirit Body can lose some of its own natural rhythm. When this occurs, one can become suicidal. If this is the case, the Spirit Body wants to free itself from the imbalance that traps it. If it cannot return to its natural flow of expansion and contraction, the Spirit cannot easily recharge itself. If this occurs, the Spirit of an individual will have an *out of body* experience, while the Spirit finds its own natural rhythm. It will then return to the Physical form and reestablish itself by stimulating the Etheric and Physical Bodies to release some of the fear and anxiety in dream form. The Spirit Body emanates light multi-colors that constantly change with each expansion and contraction. There is never a *single* color at one time.

The condition of this body depends largely on rejuvenation from the Cosmos, or its connection with the Higher Mind and Soul Bodies. However, a good connection with the Etheric and Physical Bodies does help as natural regenerator for this body. When there is harmony in these three bodies, the Spirit Body is rejuvenated. Unfortunately, most of the time, the Spirit Body is often exhausted after having frequently tried to harmonize with the lower bodies without success. It is the goal of the Spirit Body to not only find joy in being in touch with everything on Earth, but also to find joy and mastery in acceptance of the human form. Its natural pathway of flow is to circle around and through the physical form, descend towards the feet and then return to the brain where spiritual inspiration manifests.

The Higher Mind Body is a very subtle body. To understand it, one must think of pure thought as an energy form in itself. Its color is a pale electric blue. When seen psychically, it is called the Holy Spirit. This electric blue color is often tinged with silver, lilac and gold. Its form appears to be constant, to the spiritual eye, but in reality, it pulsates on such a fast vibration, that it is impossible to see. When it flows around the human form, it can be likened to an electrical current. It is only visible to the human brain. Electrical impulses stimulate the brain constantly. The nervous system is a direct receptor for the Higher Mind Body.

All that is known in the Oneness flows through every individual nerve cell. Then, knowledge is dissipated into the Etheric Body as its energy flows around the Human form. Every cell is stimulated to function primarily to survive. It is hoped that survival by circumstances will awaken that individual to a spiritual understanding of their connection with the one and all that we call God. Within this Higher Mind, energy flow is all the wisdom one needs to survive. The energy of this body flows like direct current. It spirals downward from the brain in a diagonal spiral through the physical form and then returns in an upward direction in an opposing diagonal spiral to the head. This body is never blocked. There is no stopping the flow of this body's energy. If necessary, it can disperse blocks in the other lower bodies by stimulating cross-reflexes. Unfortunately, most human beings are unaware of this natural present from God, which allows them to rejuvenate at any time.

The Soul Body, Like the Higher Mind body, is a highly refined source of energy. However, unlike the Higher Mind Body, this body does contract and expand. It reflects the dark and light of the universe. Its form is energy that is created from the constant battle between being passive or active. This body is like a clock, constantly ticking. Each tick is a self-winding generator. It can never wear out as it has continuous momentum. The refined energy of the Soul Body flows in a downward direction into the Higher Mind Body as a pure energy source. It vibrates against the Higher Mind's energy flow of direct current causing a discharge that stimulates this body to seek further awareness.

The Soul Body also affects the Spirit Body, by strengthening its vibration. This awakens the deep-subconscious mind of an individual to accept their Spirit's needs while in the body. The result is development in conscious awareness as that individual goes about their daily business.

The ultimate intention is that that individual will grow spiritually and feel connected to God. The Soul Body does not have an ascending flow. It returns to the source that is God through the Spirit Body.

The Soul Body can be seen in moments of spiritual awareness. It is usually predominantly golden, with traces of silver, copper and pink. It is capable of flaring in a pulsating manner away from the Physical Body. Its pulsation can effect a person many feet away from the individual who sends it. This type of energy can create miracles.

Angels Are Beautiful Too!

In the Spirit World, my Spirit Guides showed me how the Spirit Body had an Etheric Body, similar to that of the Earthly Etheric Body. Each emotion they felt, accompanied with each thought, had an effect on this body. By watching them, I learned to understand just how powerful this Etheric Body was, both in the flesh and in Spirit. It provided an open record of all that that individual was, had been, or hoped to become. I saw how their Spirit Body emanations fluctuated as they talked with me. I watched their colors within their Aura change like flickering lights in the darkness. They were truly angels. I saw their light and I knew that I was just as bright as they were. For the first time in my life I knew my own true beauty. I could actually feel myself radiating light quite naturally, whether or not I was healing someone. You too can radiate this great beauty!

What Holds You Together And Make You Tick!

If you've ever seen a Catherine Wheel (pinwheel) firework, then you will have an idea of what a Chakra looks like when it is fully functioning. The energy flows of these Five Bodies are both held together and controlled by the rotation of the Chakras. There are seven Major Chakras, and four pairs of Minor Chakras as well as hundreds of Mini Chakras, known as *Acu points*. Each Chakra rotates in a clockwise direction *(See diagrams at the end of this book)*.

The speed of the rotation of each individual Chakra depends on the state of harmony between the Five Bodies. If a person is negative and depressed, the Chakras slow down their rotations. When the speed of rotation slows, the individual is incapable of defending self from absorbing further negative energy. If you think of an air fan and its rotation at top speed, any paper thrown at it will be pushed away by the force of the air coming from the rotation. When it slows down, there is no air resistance and so the paper can fly through the fan. When a Chakra is rotating well, any negative energy is automatically repelled.

Each Chakra is cone shaped, with the wide mouth at the front, and the narrow end at the back of the body. Each Chakra is divided into five sections. The front part controls the flow of energy in the Physical Body. The second part controls the flow of energy in the Etheric Body. The midsection of the Chakra controls the flow of energy of the Spirit Body. The fourth section controls the flow of energy of the Higher Mind Body and the last section that of the Soul Body.

Because the last three bodies are of a more refined energy form and not of earthly vibration, they need smaller rotation impulses which stimulate them to flow at a faster rate compared with the Physical and Etheric Bodies where the energy is denser and therefore needs more push. This is like riding a bicycle up hill in first and second gear. As each Chakra rotates, energy from each body spills over and flows along the cone into the next body, thus integrating and stimulating growth in awareness.

Within each Chakra is an inner *central core* where energy is rotated and pulsed through in an ebb and flow, clockwise direction from front to rear and from rear to font, creating a double helix equal to the DNA strand. In each central core all experiences of physical, emotional, mental and spiritual nature are harmonized, resulting in a shift in the flow of the Five Bodies. All vortices surrounding each central core rotate in a similar way, but at different speeds, rather like an old fashioned clock, where accuracy creates an active and positive flow of energy, which in turn rejuvenates the Whole Being.

These inner vortices respond to physical, emotional and mental reactions to stimuli. The magnitude of the experience along with the exchange of energy from outside forces causes these inner vortices to rotate faster.

You Can Touch And Feel Your Chakras

The Seven Chakras are located as follows. The Base Chakra, (Sometimes called the Root Chakra) is between the legs over the front and rear passages with the narrow part ending just above the Heart. All old unlearned lessons are stored as energy in this Chakra. There are three vortices surrounding the central core of this Chakra. One each for physical, emotional and mental lessons derived from your experiences. Put your hand on it gently and feel your energy in this area. You hand will get warm and tingly.

Moving up the body is the Solar Plexus Chakra. This is the largest of all the Chakras. Here, energy is expelled and absorbed as human contact and/or dialogue occurs. This is the way we test ourselves by learning to interact with others. Through this Chakra, our fears, anxieties, pain and guilt are manifested, as well as our senses of love, pleasure and happiness, stimulated by our intellect from learned experiences. There are six vortices surrounding the central core within this Chakra. One each for, the Lower Self in physical, emotional and mental senses and one each for, the Higher Self, physical, emotional, mental spiritual senses. These Higher and Lower Selves are united by the fast rotation of the central core. Try feeling someone in the room with your stomach, then putting your hands over it and watching the changes that you feel.

Above the Solar Plexus Chakra is the Heart Chakra, which lies over the Heart with its center at the Sternum. Here true feelings are assimilated. All negative and positive experiences in the body generate emotions that affect the awareness of each human being.

Within this Chakra are sixteen vortices. There are five vortices each for the Lower (physical), Higher (Spiritual) and Highest (Soul) Selves that are held together by the central core, which acts as a kingpin. The basic emotions of the lower self are Fear, Pain, Anger, Guilt, and Love/Loneliness. In the Higher self, they are Fear, Trust, Faith, Love and Unity. In the Soul Body, the fears are Ascension, Descension, Separation, Assimilation and Universal (unconditional) love.

Within each category are varieties of both negative and positive emotions. On Earth, the Spirit of each individual must learn through physical experiences to understand their negative emotions and to awaken to their inner fears that manifest from the Spirit. The Spirit, when out of body has more awareness of its Soul Fears. These fears will be explained later in the book. Soul Fears cause the Spirit to search for the truth in all it touches. Ascension occurs through spiritual emotions of acceptance. Both the Lower Self-emotions and the Higher Self-emotions must interact within the center core to erase judgment. Sit with a loved one and watch how you feel one another with this Chakra. You'll feel warm and cuddly, with a growing sense of trust.

The Throat Chakra lies over the thyroid gland. Its function is to balance all that we think or speak. This Chakra is often out of balance and possibly blocked by wrong thinking and speaking. Within this Chakra are thirty-six vortices that integrate communication among Self, Higher Self and others. In this Chakra, energies of the Five Bodies mix to stimulate exchange on all levels. There are eleven vortices each for the mind, emotions and spiritual consciousness. These thirty-three vortices are harmonized by the remaining three that entwine and integrate during all aspects of communication, becoming one strong central core. This flow of energy causes vocal harmonic tones to reverberate throughout the Physical Body.

Blocked Throat Chakras cause discords that eventually manifest illness. In other words, it is important to always speak the truth.

The Third Eye Chakra lies between the brows. It is within a part of the brain that has extra-sensory perception. This Chakra, though much smaller than the rest, is filled with seventy-two vortices. Twelve of these vortices are dedicated to spiritual awareness. They are often activated in meditation or in moments of fear or great joy when the individual is in a state of momentary hypnosis. The remaining sixty vortices are dedicated to the five senses of the Physical Body. Twelve each for touch, sight, hearing, taste and smell. . All vortices entwine creating a central core that harmonizes perception in the brain.

As an individual perceives himself and his experiences, this Chakra functions to balance these impressions. It works closely with the physical workings of the Cerebellum, Cerebrum, Pineal Gland, Pituitary Gland and Medulla Oblongata. When the Third Eye Chakra is functioning well, inspiration from the Spirit Body can be transferred into the sub-conscious and conscious minds by the twelve spiritual vortices. These vortices rotate at a faster rate, causing a change in the Lower Self-vibration, which affects the flow of the energies of the Five Bodies. Perceptions can take the form of clear photo images.

Usually, this connection is made while in a dream state. If an individual is in doubt about himself or his perceptions, confusion and possible insanity may result. You may like to try sitting in a meditative state and gazing at people you know. Watch and see if you see something that you have never noticed before about them. You may even see their Auras.

The Crown Chakra has one hundred and forty four vortices. Each vortex controls one of the neural pathways of the brain and is capable of receiving and modulating the energy flow of any of the Five Bodies. At this time in Mankind's evolution, little is known about the workings of the brain or of the spiritual effect on this organ. My own experience in overcoming Parkinson's Disease, led me to understand a little more about the way I think, program my responses and select by way of being. These vortices in the Crown Chakra are all interactive and constantly entwining energy between the Physical, Etheric, Spirit, Higher Mind and Soul Bodies. These vortices control the voluntary and involuntary neuromuscular systems on a cellular level. However, eleven of these vortices are directly linked into God and The Oneness. Of the remaining hundred and thirty three vortices, seven elongated vortices are directly connected along the neuro-spine to the Base Chakra, while the remaining are used in processing an individuals entire life's experience, which is filtered back through the central core of the brain.

Crystal Acupuncture^sm is an excellent therapy to stimulate these vortices, which will indirectly or directly affect the way you think and feel. Old memories can be accessed to release pain, anger, fear and guilt along with any other emotional distress. It is always wonderful to feel connected with God and Spirit Guides, so spend time in meditation and prayer and watch what happens to you. You'll feel lighter and safer, even happier.

The Spleen Chakra lies over the spleen organ, which is situated below the ribs at the left rear of the body and extends to the right front of the body. It is slightly wider at the front of the body and has fifteen vortices within it. There are three for each of the Five Bodies. Each vortex rotates at its own speed relative to the body's energy force. These energy forces generally integrate into one vortex that forms the "core" of the Chakra. This central core has two entwined double helices rotating in opposite direction within it. One double helix rotates in a clockwise direction for balancing of the Lower Self and the other double helix rotates in an anticlockwise direction for balancing the Higher Self. These two overlapping double helices create an ebb and flow wave effect that stimulates the other Chakras to balance. Each Chakra's central core then adapts and in turn rotates at a different speed. In this way the Mind, Body and Spirit harmonize.

Vortices within each Chakra are capable of mixing the energies of the Lower Self with that of the Higher Self but without a master control there would be chaos. The Spleen Chakra is the master control that harmonizes all energies generated from mental, emotional, physical and spiritual elements of our experience. The importance of the Spleen Chakra should not be ignored during any balancing/healing process.

Those who do not listen to their inner voice and correct their way of thinking, acting or feeling, may ultimately find themselves becoming ill with such illnesses as Diabetes, or liver and spleen complaints. To cure these kinds of maladies, a radical change has to occur. Using Crystal

Acupuncture^{sm} and Teragram^{sm} Therapies daily, along with good counseling are necessary. You can test your Spleen Chakra by watching your reactions to thoughts that conjure up your imagination. If you become fearful and unstable, then your Spleen Chakra needs balancing.

Love Yourself As You Would Love Others

The Minor Chakras are in the elbows, palms, knees and center of the bottom of the feet. The Palm and Foot Chakras have cones that are wider at the surface of the body, narrowing within to the back of the hand and the top of the foot. The Knee and Elbow Chakras are wide at the kneecap and elbow joint, narrowing to the back of the leg and inside of the arm. Within each of these chakras are four vortices. There are one each for the Physical Body and its actions; the Mind and its nervous reactions; the Emotions and subsequent affects and Spirit for its experiences that cause a reaction in the physical form.

Each vortex is capable of receiving, or transmitting energy to and from the physical form. These vortices are constantly in use during any exchange with others, whether they are physical beings or spiritual ones. Psychometry is constantly being used through these Minor Chakras. Watch how your hands and feet feel when you are with others. They may be hot and sticky or cold and clammy. Maybe you are healing someone or are afraid of him or her and feel you don't belong.

These Minor Chakras are very important. We need to use them productively when we take up space and work in this world. You must be able to stand your ground or share yourself with others.

Do You Have A Thick Skin?

The Mini Chakras are, in reality, the same as Acu points in Acupuncture. Each point is a minute sensory vortex. It is said that there are over 400 points in the body, but my research has suggested that there are far more. These vortices are constantly rotating as energy passes through them. Each vortex is affected by energy from all Five Bodies. When Crystal Acupuncture^{sm} is applied to any of these points, energy can be stimulated, retarded, toned and balanced or released. These mini chakras are constantly overworked when one is emotionally, mentally and physically exhausted.

Tension and stress build and eventual blockages occur. When this happens, we become numb. We don't feel others. We only feel our own pain. Crystal Acupuncture^{sm} should be used regularly to balance the Yin and Yang energy of the human form.

Is There A Storm Brewing Inside You?

Over the years, my Spirit Guides taught me about the vortices within the Chakras. Each vortex has a freedom of its own. It can rotate at its own speed oblivious of the others and their rotation. Each vortex is akin to a tornado. If an individual is spiritually weak, the spiritual vortex will bend and distort somewhere in the middle of its form. This incorrect energy flow begins to flow back on itself causing a lack of flow in the Etheric and Physical bodies. When all vortices in one Chakra are deformed, then this Chakra is virtually useless. Negative and positive energies from outside the body are sucked into the human form. Pressure is then laid upon the other Chakras to rebalance, while the Spleen Chakra becomes overworked.

Energy arcs and sparks in all directions. Motor neurons fail to get the correct messages. The brain becomes scattered and then it desperately tries to escape the onslaught of trauma that arises with each electrical explosion. Emotional pressure generates an increase in the frequency of energy discharges that ultimately creates an electrical storm. If the environment and emotional and mental conditions of an individual's life do not change, then eventually deterioration of the other Chakras' vortices will follow along with deterioration of the brain. Such diseases as Cancer, M.S. and Alzheimer's can manifest.

Take Time Out And Then Re-Connect.

During the years that I was learning to reprogram myself with positive beliefs and ideas, I learned of the power of the brain, and the neuro-pathways that can be changed simply by redirecting thoughts while using Crystal Acupuncture^{sm}. It is possible to change the whole outlook of one's life and the way one lives. Though the vortices of the brain impulse at a different rate from those of the lower Chakras, each vortex does create an electrical impulse that causes energy to flow among all Five Bodies. They are in themselves assimilators of information from all levels of consciousness and from all levels of spirituality from both earthly and heavenly experiences.

Chakras can be rebuilt and balanced with Teragram^{sm} Therapy. Crystal Acupuncture^{sm} can redirect the energy through the chakras at the correct frequency of vibration. When all Five Bodies and chakras are in harmony, the intestines begin to gurgle.

Raising the Kundalini will also realign the chakras with one another. However, this is not advised because more harm than good can result if the mental and emotional states are not grounded and balanced. It takes years of preparation to raise the Kundalini successfully. When it occurs, hundreds of geometrical shapes and colors can be seen to pour out at the Crown Chakra. At such a time, there is ascension within that individual's vibration, which results in a revelation and a change in heart.

CHAPTER 7

The Soul Factors In Healing

No One's A Fool Really, You Made A Plan!

Everyone talks about their past lives or their "Déjà vu" experiences, but few stop to think why awareness of these arises in the first place. Deep within our brain is a true memory of who we are and where we have been before this time. Conditioning prevents us, however, from bringing this information to the surface. Besides, if you could recall everything about yourself, you would be so overloaded with information, that you would immediately enter a state of hypnosis. If you could recall all the details about every day of your life in this time, you would always be in hypnosis.

We can only cope with so much information at one time. Now, if I asked you to think of all the mistakes you have made in this life and to correct them immediately by awakening to your full awareness as an all-knowing Spirit individual, would you not be afraid of yourself and your power? Of course, you would! Your first fear to arise would be in the form of a question: "What would I do with all this powerful wisdom?" The second question would be: "What if I misuse it?" The third question would probably be, "How shall I use it?"

Before we proceed further into understanding how Crystal Acupuncture^{sm}

and Teragram^{sm} Therapies work, it is important to know that each person is encoded with a *Soul Structure*. Whenever I wanted to have control over my life or anyone else's, my Spirit Guides were always ready to point out to me that I would have to master my Soul Structure first! This Soul Structure gives each individual their unique personality and focus on their journey through life.

While I do not intend to explain the Soul Structure in detail in this book, I do advise that students obtain a copy of my book, *The Rejection Syndrome*. Further study with my Spirit Guides took me on a long journey with each client that came to see me. More and more, I saw how the Soul Structure was a brilliant piece of engineering. Once chosen, it designs our personality and character and ensures that we complete our mission to learn about others and ourselves.

Be Not Afraid!

Within the Soul Structure are Soul Fears. Each Soul Fear governs the way an individual reacts on Earth. Each Soul Fear is in itself, a lesson. These Soul Fears are:

- Fear of Ascension, which translates into the *fear of success*
- Fear of Descension, which translates into the *fear of failure*
- Fear of Separation, which translates into the *fear of independence*
- Fear of Assimilation, which translates into the *fear of losing control*
- Fear of Unconditional Love, which translates into the *fear of judgment.*

In the Universal sense, each fear has a purpose for the Spirit. These are:

- Ascension: fear of being God
- Descension: fear of being discarnate
- Separation: Fear of annihilation
- Assimilation: Fear of Power
- Unconditional Love: Fear of Surrender

Each of these Soul Fears may be encoded into the Soul Structure, but only one or two are usually used in one life. Old souls may use three or four, while ancient souls may use all five to awaken themselves to their spiritual consciousness. Generally speaking, most of us are too busy surviving in our every day lives to be able to handle more than two at one time.

These Soul Fears are most effective when used in their natural pairs. Ascension versus Descension causes a pull in one or the other direction. If one is spiritually focusing on the Fear of Success, then usually the conscious mind will focus on what is wrong, while an individual considers the pitfalls of failure. The more they focus on their failure, the more they miss their success opportunities. These people procrastinate.

Those that are mentally focusing on their success, rarely notice their failures. These people are spiritually drawn to help those who fail, in order to appreciate their success and through connecting with those who fail, learn about their own shortcomings. Whichever way you look at it, these Soul Fears force an individual to look at their fear of love. On Earth, many find their relationships falling apart because of these two Soul Fears. If both Soul Fears are encoded in the Soul Structure, then that person will have a tug of war going on within himself. These two fears cause that individual to focus on the Fear of Unconditional Love, a Soul Fear. To be in a relationship without judgment is the ideal, but usually, individuals find it hard to trust themselves or their partners.

The second pair of Soul Fears, Separation and Assimilation, also creates a tug of war within, which ultimately causes that individual to seek the understanding of their need for love. Of course, that leads them back to the Soul Fear of Unconditional Love. The battle between being able to be alone and independent versus the need to be involved and the center of attention causes individuals to search for their niche in life and to demonstrate their experiences as leaders. Often those they attract are in the mirror image of him/herself and are, therefore, in constant competition. This struggle to be recognized leads them to discover the reality that we are all the same.

The Soul Fear of Separation, when used on its own, will stimulate an individual to seek constant support, while reveling in many fears and anxieties in an effort to belong. This earthly negativity ultimately forces that individual to find his independence within the social structure without need for support. Those using the Soul Fear of Assimilation only, focus on their privacy. They will constantly look for ways to be alone to protect themselves from having to share. These people will ultimately learn to open up and join in with the crowd, while realizing that they are no better or worse than any other.

The Soul Fear of Unconditional love is often used as a subtle influence in a life. It is rarely used on its own. When it is, that individual will be exceedingly vulnerable and sensitive to the environment and his status in life. These people usually find it hard to live in a world of judgment. They often come into form for a short duration, in which time they give as much love as is humanly possible to those they encounter. These individuals often die in childhood. The few that reach adulthood usually withdraw into themselves or find seclusion, away from the maddening crowd. If this Soul Fear is used as the primary focus in conjunction with one or more of the other Soul Fears, then that individual will be very sensitive but able to live a full life. During their life, they will develop conscious awareness of themselves and evolve spiritually.

All these Soul Fears can be worked on and overcome with the use of Crystal Acupuncture℠ and Teragram℠ Therapy combined. Counseling is essential in helping each individual to see the conditioned patterns of their mind and the subsequent emotional turmoil that occurs. By deprogramming negative conditioning, these Soul Fears can be balanced and harmonized within the physical form.

For further information about conditioning, please read my books, *The Rejection Syndrome* and *The Way to Oneness.* In each of these books, you will learn how the Soul Structure and the Soul Fears are connected to the collective consciousness of the Complete Ascended Soul. The Ascended Soul is the source of divine inspiration and love.

I'll Give My Right Arm To Help You!

We have many such sayings and you ought to be careful when you use them. Maybe you really will give that right arm away. Or, maybe you'll argue with yourself and have a tug of war. Who's right, who's wrong? Which part of you is right?

It is generally accepted that one's left side is feminine, which is known as Yin energy, while the right is masculine, known as Yang. I should like to take you behind this belief and explain why we are in fact more complicated than we realize. In reality, each person's body can be divided into four parts. These four parts are receptive to the vibration of the Universe and the Higher Ascended Soul fragments that are known as Spirit Guides, Angels and the like.

These four parts are both opposing and supporting the way an individual's life is lived. Imagine yourself divided down the middle into two parts. The left side is your sensitive Feminine Self, which is more acutely aware of your emotions and of your spirit. The Right side is your Masculine Self, which is more directly concerned with the way you use your time on Earth. Now imagine that these two parts have been cut laterally separating the back from the front. The front part of your body is the Masculine Self, while the back part of your body is the Feminine Self.

Now that you can imagine yourself in four parts, visualize the left rear part. Know that this section of your body is extra sensitive because it is doubly feminine, very spiritually emotional and highly inspirational. This part of yourself is controlled by your Spirit's desires to live a life that will allow it to ascend in consciousness. This part of yourself is where you find your intuitive, knowing self and your sense of spiritual love along with strength and power to continue, despite the odds.

As you visualize your front left side of your body, you will note that it is both masculine and feminine. However, the masculine part rules. Here your soft loving part of your Higher Feminine Self blends from the rear into your Lower Feminine Self which in turn blends with your Lower Masculine Self. This causes a mellowing of your strong aggressive Masculine Self, which results in a shift in consciousness that allows your Spiritual Self to connect from the rear. This creates an emotional desire to change in some way.

The right rear part of your body is also both feminine and masculine. Here the Higher Feminine part rules. Your Spiritual Self causes your Masculine Self to question the material choices that you made. By searching through data, your brain is able to access a crosscurrent of energy that is created between the left front and right rear parts of your body. In this way, you challenge yourself to find the harmony between your thoughts, emotions and deeds.

The right front part of your body is doubly masculine. Here action is the main focus. Everything you decide to do is logically worked out and then challenged by the left rear part of your body that is doubly feminine. Your brain accesses this crosscurrent exchange of energy, which results in your ability to double-check yourself to make sure that your spirit is following the right pathway.

By connecting with all the right physical things that become tools to experiment with, you learn to grow spiritually. Your brain learns to read the signals from these four parts of your body and then to create memory in a cross-reference form. Eventually, it is hoped that you will achieve clarity of mind and harmony of emotions with a sense of spiritual elation and awareness.

Get Connected!

The four parts of your body help manifest your cross reflexes in the nerves. If you do not listen to your Higher Self (Spirit), or if you are not aware of your true thoughts and emotions, then you will probably become sick. There is no justification in keeping up old habits that cause illness, so get connected and let energy flow.

If the left front side of your body is well connected to the left rear side of your body, then many talents and subsequent emotional lessons will manifest which result in a spiritual awakening. This will help you to get a healthy body with good energy flow along the meridians. In like manner, if the right front side of your body is well connected to the right rear part, then you will have a good outlook on life with practical application of your ideas. You will, as a result, manifest your hopes and desires. When you get active, healing and rejuvenation occurs because of a good energy flow along the meridians.

Be Your Own Protector.

Try to find a balance within that will allow your Yin/Yang energy to harmonize. Your Female Self must nurture your Male Self, while your

Male Self must protect your Female Self. Ultimately, you must become lovingly wise, and wisely loving!

Many diseases are caused by an imbalance between these four parts of the body. Crystal Acupuncture^{sm} will stimulate your meridians and move blocked energy, which will result in an awareness of the changes you need to make. Though fear may manifest, counseling and Teragram^{sm} Therapy follow up sessions will enable you to touch your Higher Self and awaken spirituality within. This of course, will help you in the rejuvenation of cells and the elimination of illness.

Here are a few of the categories of disorders that can be reduced or released completely:

- *Various Diseases caused by Muscular/ Nervous/ Mental/ Emotional conditioning.*
- *Deterioration of organs and systems caused by fear, pain, anger and guilt: Digestive/Glandular/Circulatory/Neuro systems*
- *Deterioration of bones, ligaments and tissue caused by anger, guilt and loneliness: Rheumatism/Arthritis/ Spinal Pain /Aches etc.*
- *Deterioration of reproductive organs caused by guilt, fear and loneliness.*
- *Deterioration of the five senses caused by fears from living environments*

Many of these illnesses are accompanied by co-dependency habits, such as sleeping pills, alcohol, illegal drugs etc.

Both Spiritual Crystal Acupuncture^{sm} and the original Crystal Acupuncture^{sm}, in conjunction with Teragram^{sm} Therapy, and Aromatherapy with Reflexology can be successfully used to move energy along the meridians. Then a consistent current of energy flow can effectively create stimulation of the cross reflexes. This creates an ebb and flow in the pulsation of the five bodies, which generally results in an inner sense of well-being. Healing follows.

CHAPTER 8

Crystal Acupuncture^sm Crystals

It has been necessary to describe to you of all the ways emotional, mental and spiritual conditioning has been coded into the physical body before proceeding with the actual understanding of the techniques. Once you begin using Crystal Acupuncture^sm, you will recognize that which has been mentioned arising in the person you are healing. In this chapter, I explain the nature of some of the crystals I selected to use that are readily available, and the techniques of applying Crystal Acupuncture^sm. However, for further information concerning the Acu Points, please refer to The Book of Crystal Acupuncture ^sm and Teragram ^sm Therapy Diagrams, in which specific illnesses and treatments are listed.

Nature's Helping Hand.

Minerals, just like everything else on this Earth, have a way of providing us with Nature's helping hand. As plants and trees provide us with medicine, food, paper, houses etc., so do rocks. The mining of various rocks has opened the world to more than just its monetary value. Rocks are now called crystals in the metaphysical world. Crystals are minerals that are conducive to the flow of human energy and the more subtle bodies.

As stated earlier in this book, I have spent years researching the effects of my energy flow on crystals and of their effect on others and myself. One of my earliest finds as a child, was natural Agate. Those brownish white stones seemed nearly always to attract me. Over the years, I learned that Agate has a natural healing vibration which, when tapped into, could create a miracle. And, like many natural healing herbs, was in abundance. Right in your back garden is a stone waiting to make you better!

Over time, I learned that Agate, Quartz, Jasper, and several other crystal stones were all members of the Chalcedony family, which harmonize body, mind, emotions and spirit. For that reason, I decided to include and use these crystals in my own Crystal Acupuncture^sm set. You should acquire your own stones and become familiar with your set. Do add new crystals from time to time and do experiment with them on yourself and on those clients who are agreeable.

I am often asked if more expensive crystals are more effective than those explained in this book. The truth is No! It is not the monetary value that makes a crystal the best healing tool on the planet, but rather where it was made. Each country has a different vibration within the land where it formed. Therefore, Agate found in Brazil, is different from Agate found in England. When different rocks form together, they create a different vibration within the area. Some areas in the world are magnetic. These areas produce good rock formations that help us polarize our energy. Other areas produce rock that is calming and relaxing, while still others stimulate and rotate energy within the human form.

Get Rid Of Garbage That Sticks!

I am sure that at some time you have found yourself sitting in a part of the world where a sense of earthly energy seemed to harmonize you and set you at peace. For example, a quiet day on a sandy beach, or in the mountains replaces positive ions with negative ions in those environments. Positive ions are particles that have dust and other "stuff" stuck to them. Their very nature is to attract all the negative "stuff" you do not need. The negative ions are reversed. Nothing sticks to them! Therefore, at the beach you find those negative ions and they make you feel better.

While I do not pretend to be anything of a scientist, I do know, through my own observations when healing that many of these positive ions are often trapped in a person's Aura. These people are usually very negative in their attitude about themselves and their life. Teragram^sm Therapy helps one to release these ions by stimulating the chakras. As each chakra rotates faster, it dispels them. Ions are held in the Aura by negative or positive polarities. Magnetic therapy can be very helpful in eliminating those wretched positive ions. However, what is a magnet? It is a mineral that has been polarized. Iron is a good conductor of energy. I'm sure many of you did school experiments with iron filings and a magnet. We ooh'd and ah'd at the shapes we could make. We could clearly see the directional flow of energy created by the shape of the iron filings.

Many of the natural healing crystals have iron composites within them, which make them useful tools in removing those unwanted ions. Just like iron, many of these stones are capable of carrying energy through them.

My research over the years has led me to understand how many of these crystals allow energy to pass through them. By trial and error, with careful attention paid to the advice from my Spirit Guides, I was able to watch a crystal and the effect it had as I used it. I found that some crystals bounced energy back and forth at a crazy rate, building up momentum within until it shot out like a laser light. Closer study revealed that that laser beam was vibrating at an extremely fast rate and has an angular appearance, rather like a line of V's joined together. Quartz's vibration causes everything in its path to vibrate also. Its effect in the human body, is to shake up trapped energy which, when moved, moves abruptly.

To understand the type of effect it can have on you, think of yourself as being enclosed in a barrel and tossed into churning water where you are tossed around inside. The barrel makes its way towards the edge and then you feel yourself falling over Niagara Falls. Everything you know to be safe is lost once you are inside that barrel. All your fears will surface. Fears from living life, to fears of death will spill out as you face yourself and the ride in the barrel over the edge. Imagine the inner peace you will find, when you survive the ordeal and realize how wonderful your life is and how brave and beautiful you are. Your ordeal will have given you a desire for more positive things in your life. You would appreciate yourself and everything you do.

Clear Quartz crystal can have this kind of effect on you. It can shake up all your old energy patterns and stimulate them to surface. It can amplify your emotions and draw you into yourself to face the truth. It will energize you and stimulate you to survive by facing your fears and erasing them. If you do not want to change, don't wear Quartz. Below are more crystals that you can use.

Sodalite is a member of the Agate family. It too can stimulate your energies to move. However, unlike the Quartz that affects all of your five bodies, Sodalite awakens the Higher Mind Body. By shaking up this body, your lower bodies are stimulated into awareness of the Higher Mind Body and its needs. This crystal's vibration is more refined than the Quartz. The rate of speed with which energy leaves the crystals is faster and less disruptive. It appears to look more like the flow of electricity. When this crystal is used, the end result is that the Physical Body feels depleted of energy. When the human form is resting, it is open in the sensory sense, to receive new impressions. Revelations can occur with use of this crystal.

Rose Quartz and Smokey Quartz, like Clear Quartz, are energizers and amplifiers, however, the way energy moves through them is circular. Energy spins round and round along the crystal and then out along the meridian in a continual rotation pattern. This rotation of energy causes the Five Bodies to harmonize and tone. Both crystals have a calming effect on the heart and circulation, as well as on the emotional and spiritual states of the Etheric and Spirit Bodies.

Amethyst, a member of the Quartz family, has a positive effect on the Spirit Body. It is far more refined than those crystals mentioned above. Its natural way of carrying energy is to spin energy passing though it. When this type of energy is passed along the meridians, it connects with the Spirit body, where it harmonizes the Spirit's energy flow. This has a calming effect on the Physical and Etheric Bodies. When the Spirit Body flows correctly, Changes occur in the Physical body, along with a change of attitude. This crystal is often seen to act as a tranquilizer.

Carnelian is both an energizer and harmonizer. I often noticed different reactions in the Physical Body while using this crystal. The natural density of this stone allows energy to find its own pathway according to the energy passing though it. It seemed to have a natural rotation as well as an undulating one. These two natural flows spiral and entwine together. The ensuing result is a rotating vibrating energy. This kind of energy affects the

Physical body in a variety of ways by affecting the Etheric Body directly. As various blocks in the Etheric Body are dispersed, the Physical Body relaxes with a release of nerve twitches and other bodily feelings. Old emotions can arise as they are released. Carnelian is, in itself, an excellent crystal for balancing the glands of the body which lie directly within the Major Chakras. Once the glands of the body function well, healing always occurs.

Hematite is an excellent crystal to help heal the mind. The mind is a power organ by itself. All your thoughts are pure energy, which passes around, back and forth in the brain. Often the energy of the brain becomes caught in a loop. The same thoughts keep arising. All those old emotions keep you ill. It has magnetic polarity properties that help the energy of the brain to find its natural pathway out of the loop. Hematite is a harmonizer and, like Amethyst, has a refined vibration rather like electricity. It flows smoothly around the meridians by simply forcing any blocks in its way to dissolve. Each body is generally affected by the wave of energy it causes as blocks are dispersed. Harmony of mind, body and spirit are the result.

Amazonite is one of my favorite crystals. It has all the properties of Quartz, Amethyst and Aventurine. Energy moves through this crystal in a rotational, undulating, refined vibration that causes the Etheric Body to release old issues around negative memories and to bring harmony from the Spirit Body into this body. As the Physical Body accepts the changes in the Etheric Body, The Spirit Body blends more positively with the Etheric Body, resulting in mental and emotional changes of attitude. In meditation or hypnosis, this stone can connect the Higher Mind and Soul Bodies, which could result in a 'miracle' healing. The Etheric Body must release all negative programming for this to occur.

Aventurine is one of the most calming crystals available. Like Jade, its form allows a slow undulating gentle pulsating energy to flow through it and on into the Physical Body. Its effect creates a sense of wellness in the physical emotions, which in turn affects the Etheric Body. Old emotions are released. As this simple vibration circulates, it slowly causes the other bodies to harmonize. New cells begin to grow within the physical form after such a healing.

Fight The Good Fight With All Your Might

Whether a crystal is vibrating, rotating, circulating or stimulating, energy is always moving around one or more of the five bodies. Whatever occurs is the result of the patient's acceptance of their need to change. No matter how good the energy of the healer is, the natural healing process can only take place if the patient is spiritually ready to change. I have often had clients who have assured me they are ready to change. They expected me to wave a magic wand and make all their pain and their lessons go away. As treatments progressed they became aggressive and started to fight against making changes. They wanted me to make it easy for them. It can't be done!

Each of us has to walk our own path and in time, each of us finds a way to heal ourselves. I am only the catalyst that helps someone to cure him/herself. The ultimate cure is the realization that the conditioned life is wrong. Fight to free your mind from entrapment. Change your mind, change your heart and connect to the Oneness and then you will have a major opportunity to overcome your illness by learning about your true self and the real reason you are here on Earth.

Each of these crystals was selected for its qualities as explained above. Here is a more detailed description of the type of effects these crystals can have on a person. My research is in agreement with Melody whose book, ***Love Is In The Earth***, I highly recommend.

AMAZONITE: "Synthesis" Gently harmonizes the Heart and Throat Chakras, and masculine and feminine energies. It aligns all Chakras and brings the user back to their "power spot." This crystal also brings all energy back into the center of the physical form. Emotionally and mentally, it gives stamina, strength of character, faith and compassion. Physically, it helps with calcium deficiency and new growth of body tissue. It is compatible with the vibration of the Fifth Chakra, the Throat, which will stimulate speech with balanced expression. This crystal is a Virgo stone, calling for perfection, serenity, and grounding of emotions that result in an acute sense of reality. It vibrates to #2 and #3 tone, which translates into the musical notes D & E in the scale of C Major.

AMETHYST: "Metamorphosis." This crystal is an ancient healer of all levels of body, mind and spirit. It cleanses, purifies, restructures and renews.

It transforms lower energies into a higher refined vibration, and protects the user against psychic manipulation. Physically, it heals bone maladies, such as arthritis, as well as stimulating the senses of hearing, smell and taste. This stone brings spiritual peace and physical contentment by freeing the Etheric Body of learned conditioning. It clears the Aura of negativity, and helps in deepening meditation states. It protects an individual from negative verbal attack as well as protecting the psychic from invasion from earthbound spirits. This stone vibrates in harmony with the Sixth Chakra, The Third Eye, and is the Pisces birthstone. It vibrates to the # 3 & # 6 tone, which is musically, E and A note of the Major key C. This crystal harmonizes your Etheric and Physical Bodies allowing you to release the watery emotions of anger and pain and be receptive to the Spirit Body's vibration of pure love. This can cause a revolution in the way you live your life.

AVENTURINE: "Healer of the Heart & Soul." This crystal balances masculine and feminine energies in the lower self. Its effect can be felt strongly in the front of the body at first. As energy moves, it can be felt in the rear too, as the Higher Self balances through the stimulation of cross-reflexes, causing a harmonizing of the Spiritual Masculine and Feminine self. The result is a development in the levels of creativity and leadership with a passion for the pleasures of life. This crystal enables one to make the right decisions and to feel as though embraced in a blanket of spiritual love. Physically, it helps heal the heart, lungs, adrenals and muscular system, which in turn aids the liver and pancreas to function effectively. In meditation, this crystal stimulates connection with the Soul Body and spiritually releases heartache from the Etheric Body. It then stimulates the emergence of true creativity with a flaming passion that motivates one towards success. It helps energy to flow throughout the reproductive system to balance male and female energies and to align all Five Bodies, creating a true state of tranquility. This crystal vibrates in harmony with the Fourth Chakra, The Heart, and is the birthstone of Aries. It vibrates in the tone of #1 and #4, which is the musical note of C and F in the C Major key.

CARNELIAN: "Ambition and Drive." This crystal inspires a positive courageous confidence. It motivates, activates and energizes personal power to manifest, which always reveals hidden talents. It protects the user from becoming lost in a sea of negative emotions, by stimulating insights and awareness that arise from the Spirit Body. It also protects the wearer from other people's negative emotional outbursts, such as envy, fear and rage. As these negative energies hit the surface of the Aura, it causes that individual to mentally re-assess self through clear and precise thinking, thus avoiding losing self in negative emotions. This crystal reminds one to be in the moment and to go with the flow.

As Carnelian stimulates the inner child to manifest in positive ways, a belief in the magic of life and the power of the Spirit is awakened with a passion. For this reason, this crystal stimulates a good connection to Spirit Guides and their world. Love abounds in self and family. Physically, this crystal balances the glands of the body, as well as the Liver, Pancreas and Spleen. Its vibration is in harmony with the Second Chakra, The Spleen, and therefore, harmonizes all the other Chakras by stimulating the second Chakra (Spleen) to balance and harmonize the five bodies. This is another Aries stone, which vibrates to the notes #1 and #3, which are the musical notes of C and E in the Major key of C.

HEMATITE: "Stone of Mental Mastery." This crystal stimulates photographic memory. Behind every picture are a thousand words, and this crystal helps you remember all you have said or heard. It brings clarity, with balance and calm reason. It dissolves negative ideas and opens channels for receptivity from The Spirit Body to receive unconditional love for self. It aids in making truly peaceful, loving relationships. It also helps to eliminate negative conditioning from the Etheric Body and induces the realization of truths that effectively slow the mind down, to make problem solving easier. New information is then easily retained. This is a good crystal to use if you are taking a study course. This crystal physically calms the nerves; erases panic symptoms, cools the body and normalizes circulation. Hematite controls fear, pain, anger and guilt, while erasing loneliness. It transforms negativity into spiritual joy and bonds the Spirit Body with The Etheric and Physical Bodies, thus preventing states of escapism, such as suicide or reclusiveness in a mental depressive state. This crystal vibrates in harmony with the Sixth, Third Eye and Seventh Crown Chakras. It's musical vibration in the Major key of C is tone #1, #2 an #7, which is C, D and top B.

QUARTZ: "Universal Conduit." This crystal is best when it is clear without rutilation. It amplifies, focuses, stores and transforms energy. It is an excellent crystal for focusing on affirmations and prayers. It stimulates psychic perception, which allows a release of negative ideas and emotions, which of course, allows one to evolve spiritually at one's own pace. This crystal can bring negative thoughts and emotions to the surface to be displayed for revision and later release. Quartz empowers and stimulates action in procrastinators. Physically, it opens all the meridians, allowing the energy of all Five Bodies to flow, which directly affects every part of the human body.

In meditation with this crystal, personal history can be erased, along with negative mindsets. This allows the lower mind and emotions of the Etheric Body to harmonize by releasing stored up unwanted energy from old memories. Subsequently, the Lower Self-perceptions can harmonize with the Higher Mind Body, bringing in inspiration and psychic development. It lifts the spirit towards love and peaceful union with God. Quartz is itself the Major Scale of C to high C inclusive. It vibrates constantly in the tones #1- #8 and is, therefore, a harmonic vibration that is considered to be the Crystal of the Spirit & Soul.

ROSE QUARTZ: "Stone of Warmth and Love." This crystal is the true balancer of the Yin and Yang energy. Female and male energy entwines to culminate in a true expression of unconditional love. This crystal helps heal emotional pain like a gentle calming salve. It opens the heart to the beauty within and without. Cherubic energies are attracted to the user, protecting, and dissolving negativity. It stimulates the Spirit Body to harmonize with the Etheric Body by stimulating inspirational ideas, full of passion and enthusiasm to over-ride negative conditions. Desire manifests, which in turn results in an opening of sexual expression and an attraction to romance and love of oneself. Physically, it clears the body of excess fluids and promotes healing by releasing tension and stress. It helps in the circulation of blood, and strengthens the lymphatic system. It vibrates in harmony with the Fourth Chakra, The Heart, and is the birthstone of Taurus and Libra. Its tone is #2 and #6 vibration, which is the musical note of D and A.

SODALITE: "Stills the mind." This crystal brings in a lightness of being by stimulating the mind to face truths that will help individuals to build good thoughts about themselves and others. It assists in the growth of self-esteem, worth and value, by releasing negativity directly connected to learned opinions and judgment. It connects the energy of the Higher

Mind Body and Soul Bodies and helps integrate them all the way into the Physical Body. Physically, it aids in sleep, cleanses the digestive system and balances the metabolic rate by stimulating the glands in the body. This crystal is also an effective harmonizer of the Etheric Body. It aids in controlling the rate of flow of energy and can be used to calm and relax the mind and the emotions, which results in a sense of wellness. Sodalite is both #5 and #7 in tone vibration, which are the musical notes of G and B in the Major key of C.

Though each crystal carries a musical tone, the human ear cannot hear it. However, my Spirit Guides inform me that this can be proved in a technical way under laboratory conditions. When the correct musical note is applied to the crystal, definite pulse energy can be felt which in turn will cause a physical reaction in an individual. Unfortunately, I do not have the equipment or the time to prove the point. I am sure someone somewhere is carrying out this experiment and if so, I would love to hear from him or her.

In the meantime, I have selected several musical compositions that resonate through the crystals while I am using them. Every healer is automatically in tune with the Major key of C while working. As their Psychic sense evolves and their healing powers increase, their sensitivity to feeling the musical notes will increase. The result is an effect in the harmonics of the healer and the patient. A blending of energies is in reality like singing in tune. A song sung well always softens the heart and lifts the vibration of an individual. Crystal Acupuncture[sm] is a powerful harmonic therapy that successfully stimulates tones and balances the energy flow of the Five Bodies.

The above descriptions for the stones and their properties reflect the wonderful knowledge and research presented in the book, *Love is in the Earth* by Melody, Copyright 1995 and published by Earth-Love Publishing House. Please refer to this wonderful work for more complete descriptions of these stones and hundreds of others that have Metaphysical properties.

CHAPTER 9

Fluff Your Aura With Crystal Acupuncture^{sm}

Painting The Aura? – Color It Gold!

As was explained in a prior chapter, your Five Bodies each have their own energy flow. These five energies form the *Aura*. People have often asked me what color their Aura is. I have to inform them that the Aura is constantly changing its color. Each body has its own color according to the way the energy flows around it. These colors vary in intensity. Collectively these colors seem to blend into one dominant color. It is like taking several colors in a paint box and mixing them up. If you have a great deal of blue, and red, then a dark purple will form. If you add yellow, then you are looking at a dark brown color.

Often, the overall color of the Aura is a mixture of predominantly negative colors in each body. When they blend, a dense dark Aura can be seen. This person will be in a great deal of pain, physically, emotionally, mentally and spiritually. A lot of work will have to be done to change their perception about themselves, their loved ones, and their purpose for living. They will need to have a change of heart and learn to trust themselves, the world and God. This is often too much to ask. Many prefer to suffer indefinitely, even to die, rather than adapt. Take a leap of faith and color your Aura gold.

Swing High, Swing Low! See Energy Flow!

You can dowse the Aura with a pendulum to find the dark places. Dense colors can be found where the Aura is weak. In these areas, polarity of the Five Bodies is often non-existent. Hold the pendulum a foot above the weak area and watch as it is pulled in towards the body, as though being sucked into a whirlpool.

Using a crystal pendulum can be exceedingly helpful. By dowsing the area of weakness with different crystals, and with attunement from the healer, energies can be felt as either attractive or repellent. If Aventurine is held over the affected area and appears to be pulled in towards the body, then this stone is polarizing with the energies of the Etheric Body. This gives the healer a clue that their patient's cure really lies in the emotions and mental attitude of the patient.

If a Rose Quartz pendulum is held over the negative part of the Aura and is drawn in, then it is safe to assume that all Five Bodies need a great deal of work done to correct their flows. This also means that Teragram[sm] Therapy should be applied to stimulate the Chakras and to rebuild the cones with each one.

If a Sodalite pendulum is held over the negative part of the Aura, and is drawn in, this provides a clear indication that the patient is suffering from inadequate mindsets created in childhood. These mindsets cause emotional turmoil within the Etheric and Spirit Bodies. Healing must be given through inspirational awareness.

The healer should be conscious of the patient's Higher Mind Body and use crystals that will stimulate energy to flow down from this body into the lower bodies. While this is done, simple counseling with alternative suggestions should be given. This may include the use of hypnosis to block out or clear old memories that have been accumulated within an obsessive mind. Regular Crystal Acupuncture[sm] treatments should be frequently carried out with follow-up sessions by a good counselor. These individuals usually need a strong support system. Try to get them connected to a help organization.

Believe What You Feel. Trust What You Know.

Other crystals can be used in similar ways to dowse the body. Whichever one you choose, allow yourself to attune to the idea of finding negativity within the patient's body. Your natural psychic self will use Psychometry to find it. When you have located one or more places in the Aura, you will find yourself wondering what is the cause. As you focus, there will be a natural response within yourself. Follow your intuition and trust. With regular practice, your psychic senses will develop. However, it is always wise to find a good teacher who can help you along your journey.

It's Time To Say 'Goodbye.

Unfortunately, negative people usually come in the company of *Lost Souls*, or e*arthbound spirits* as they are often called. These spirits are individuals who have died and are still seeking earthly help. Their Spirit is considered discarnate, resulting from abuse of their last earthly life. If you find yourself sensing that you are dealing with a form of mild possession, then it will be necessary to protect yourself from negative invasion. Closing your Chakras is most important. Please take time to read my book *The Way to Oneness* or find other books that will teach you how to protect yourself.

An immediate way of protecting yourself is to be conscious of your Spirit Body and, while in prayer, to attune to your Higher Self and Guides for guidance. Also, remember to think often of golden light surrounding you. This golden light is of a high vibration, which forces any earthbound spirits to ascend into heaven (spirit world) or, if it is their wish, to leave the room.

Do not rush into the idea of explaining possession to your friend/patient/client. They may be frightened or see you as some sort of idiot. Simply teach them how to close their own Chakras and to walk in the golden light. This should do the trick. If you have an extreme case of possession, where that person is unable to separate him/herself from a spirit, you will need to seek the advice of an exorcist, such as a priest. Do not get into hocus-pocus rituals. Usually, the earthbound spirit wants to be rescued.

By talking quietly about releasing the client/patient from the earthbound spirit's possession, the spirit will feel itself losing hold, as that individual awakens to the idea that they are not making decisions for themselves.

Once each realizes their individuality, separation will quite naturally occur. God's Law of Karma, "No one fragment shall invade the space of another, on any level, in any dimension" will fall into effect. All five laws are explained in my book *The Way to Oneness*.

If you find yourself worrying about having to deal with such a client - Don't! You do not want to attract that kind of person. Be positive and simply focus on helping those in need. Trust that your Spirit Guides will keep you safe from harm and only bring you those that are the right people for you to heal. If you get a possession case, then it's time for you to find out what you really know from your own spirit consciousness or maybe from another therapist who does this kind of work.

Sensing Change Is Becoming Gloriously Happy.

Before you carry out any form of healing, you should remember to connect to your higher vibrations in the form of prayer/meditation and ask your client/patient to do the same. Then ask them to release as much negative energy as is possible, by visualizing their negative energy going into the ground, where Mother Nature neutralizes that energy. You should do likewise while standing quietly to one side. Then both you and the client/patient should be open and receptive to receiving connection from God and Spirit Guides to help in the healing process.

The most common question any of my clients ask me about Crystal Acupuncture[sm] is "What will I feel, and how will I know it's working?" Those that are Physical types and are use to watching and feeling their bodies move will have no problem feeling the crystal's effects. The bottom line is, you will feel all kinds of sensations, such as itches, tickles, pinches, sharp and subtle pains, twitches, rumbles, flinches, static electrical sensations, sudden reflex jumps, and more.

During our lives, we have had too numerous physical sensations to mention here. All of them have an emotional and mental meaning to the brain, so as these physical sensations occur, pictorial images, along with emotions can arise into the conscious mind. If this is the case, memories should be observed and then unconditionally released. Getting lost in a memory and the emotion can cause a back flow and resistance to crystal healing. On a conscious level, it can create an obsession.

If this is the case, simply have the client/patient repeat to him/herself "I release this history," Then instruct them to take deep breaths, which will allow energy to flow on through to the nearest Chakra where it will be re-balanced. When a release is completed, new programming in the form of simple statements spoken aloud is highly effective. The voice creates tones, which have resonance that stimulates energy to move. This energy is then stored in the cellular-neuro-muscular memory.

Effective statements to have your client/patient repeat aloud are: "I am positive." "I am happy." "I am strong." "I can do anything." "I love myself very much." Follow each statement with direction that the client/patient feel these statements emotionally and then to focus on sensing how energy from this thought is changing the Physical Body. Encourage them to feel how energy is flowing around their body, giving each cell a new neuro-muscular memory. During this time you can use Crystal Acupuncture^{sm} to tone and balance the energies of the Five Bodies. When this is done, rebuild the Chakras where necessary with the use of Teragram^{sm} Therapy.

Crystal Acupuncture^{sm} Techniques

My methods of use of each crystal are mentioned in The Book of Crystal Acupuncture ^{sm} and Teragram ^{sm} Therapy Diagrams, but for practical purposes, I have chosen to include and augment them in this book.

Impound (Stimulate). Apply firm pressure of the tip of the crystal into the acupuncture point and then a quick release. This should be done in a rhythmic pattern several times. This forces blocked energy to move.

On several occasions, I noticed some of my students impounding their points as though they were trying to drill a hole in their thumb and at such a rapid rate, that it caused their Aura to pulsate and shiver. This kind of extreme movement is not necessary. A gentle push of the point into the thumb with a simple slow in and out rhythm in keeping with the second hand of your watch is sufficient. Rapid movement is only necessary in extreme cases, where the client is very blocked and extremely ill emotionally, mentally and physically, and radical treatment is needed. Radical treatment causes a heavy emotional release. Treatment should include follow up sessions and close attention should be given in one hour separate counseling sessions at least twice a week.

For a normal release, the Acu point should be impounded five or six times. Then the crystal should be held still on the point allowing healing energy to flow through the crystal. During that time, the therapist should watch for physical changes in breathing pattern and bodily reactions. If none occur, repeat the impounding technique. Once you have a response, holding the crystal on the Acu point with slight pressure will begin the toning/balancing process.

Toning/Balancing. The therapist should allow the energy to flow through the crystals and out into the client. It will then flow around the meridians and back to the therapist. When this is done the therapist will feel an electrical sensation in the hands. Some physical therapists may feel energy changes within their own body, as they adapt to the healing process and their client's shift in energy.

Releasing excess negative energy. The point of the crystal is rotated in a clockwise direction on the acupuncture point. Do not spin the crystal. Do this in the same manner as drawing a period on a piece of paper. This creates energy in a spiral flow that causes energy levels in all the Five Bodies to integrate creating a harmonic shift. During this time, a client may move into hypnosis and may have an emotional outburst or physical response, such as a sudden jump as though in shock.

Read The Signs!

Use your senses to see yourself, or if you are the therapist and psychic, it is possible to see a shift in each body as they align their energies. While impounding the crystal, you may see clouds of white, blue and various sparkling explosions of color along with red and green leaving the Aura. Dark colors of varying hues may also be seen as spiral forms leaving the Aura. While you are toning and balancing, expect to see sparkles of white, yellow, lilac and various pinks as each body finds its own energy flow.

When releasing occurs, you may see that the Aura often looks white as all bodies blend into one, because all colors mix to create white. Further observation will reveal to you an electric blue color that entwines the white.

This electrical blue color is the primary color of the Spirit Body. You may see gold following around the Aura, particularly around the head of the client during this amalgamation. The treatment is then finished for the day.

The Intellectual Type.

If you or the client is an "Intellectual" type, then you/he/she will not need to feel their bodies adapting. You or they will be lost within thoughts trying to understand what is happening. Many of these thoughts will surface as a result of the energy changes that are occurring in the Five Bodies. During treatment these types often fall into a hypnotic sleep. While sleeping, they will have physical responses just the same as the "Physical" type. These responses may be less demonstrative, but are visible. If you are the therapist, then you should look for *ideo-motor responses*, (neuro-muscular triggers: flinches) in the face, hands and feet. Do not worry if it does not happen too often.

Trust your instincts and let yourself feel what is happening psychically. "Intellectual" types are often easier to help. Self-help is possible. Once in a hypnotic state, you/they will readily accept any positive suggestions for change that are given. On a conscious level, "Intellectual" types simply rationalize that changes need to be made and then make them without thought or need to get closure. They have the ability to walk away from their past.

The Physical Type

"Physical" types find it hard to adapt. They are constantly looking for closure from every situation they find themselves in. They are emotionally attached to everything and want to be totally understood as well as to receive full recognition for their suffering before they can let go. Hypnotic statements are accepted, but these positive statements are often blocked by rationalizations beginning with "but…," Counseling is very important for these types who love to talk out their problems.

Healing Can Take No Time At All!

There is no set time allotted for each placement of the crystal and the time of use on that point. Application of Crystal Acupuncture^{sm} is entirely dependent on intuition in self or the healer and the client. Each client, in his or her own time, will release negative energy. The therapist must be patient and give the client time to react to each stage of the treatment. When the treatment is completed on an Acu point, gently massage it, allowing it to integrate back into the flow.

Follow The Flow.

In The Book of Crystal Acupuncture^{sm} and Teragram^{sm} Therapy Diagrams, there are many diagrams showing the Acu points that should be used in dealing with specific problems. However, over the years I have found that Crystal Acupuncture^{sm} applied to the feet or hands only, can be just as effective. Each toe is connected to the thumb/fingers on the same side of the body. Left big toe meridian flows up through the center of the body to the head and then down the arm to the left thumb. The second toe meridian flows up the body to the left of the big toe meridian and then on down to the index finger. The middle toe meridian flows up over the nipples and temples and then down the arm to the middle finger. The forth toes meridian flows up the left side of the body and connects with the third tow meridian. It then flows back down the inside of the arm to the fourth finger. The fifth toes meridian flows up the body to the heart and on to the head and then back down through the elbow to the little finger.

All major meridians flow up and down the front and back of the body. Each meridian is connected to other minor meridians, providing alternative routes for energy to flow, rather like driving a car across America. You can take the Highways and the Byways and eventually arrive at your destination. The longer the journey, the more tired you are likely to be. If your energy is not flowing well along the meridians and has to find a detour, then you will most definitely feel unwell.

Replenish And Rejuvenate Regularly.

Even the fittest and most balanced people need to refresh their meridians from time to time. A Crystal Acupuncture^{sm} treatment can be very rejuvenating. Crystal Acupuncture^{sm} treatments should not be given more than twice a week. This allows time for changes in the energy flow to manifest in daily life. A client must have time to face old problems and find a new way to deal with them. Sometimes it is necessary for them to encounter a situation that will be, in itself, a 'button-pusher'. These 'button-pushers' are very important. They allow old emotions to surface. Here is an example. A client has a deep emotional block to do with old childhood anger. Crystal Acupuncture^sm has stimulated this anger and brought it to the surface. Now the client is at home and ready to have their button pushed. He/she is asked to do something simple and suddenly finds him/herself being uneasy and angry. They have a sudden outburst and in a child-like manner scream and shout and generally lose any sense of control. Anger is then released along with child-like sobs etc. At this point, the client needs to notice him/herself and acknowledge their release. Awareness will arise in the following hours that will allow the client to understand what they have learned through this outburst.

An example might be that, as a child, they wanted their own way and learned that they could not have it; so they made a primary tape stating: "Don't try to get anything. You can't have it unless it's given to you first." The new realization will be: "I can go get everything I want myself."

Some releases are less obvious. Dreams can often help an individual to overcome negativity with new positive ideas. Creative pursuits can open up new ways to evolve. There are many general things that can happen to the client following a Crystal Acupuncture^sm treatment. It is often advisable to have a diary in which to keep a record of the mental and emotional changes that occur while carrying on with one's normal daily routines.

A few individuals never notice the effect of their changes. They just seem to find a way to break the ties that bind them. They are often spiritually awakened and in the habit of looking for ways to improve and are therefore adaptable. Unfortunately, most of us fight ourselves with guilt and loneliness.

Any Time, Anywhere, Use Your Crystals.

Whatever the type of person you are. Crystal Acupuncture^sm will help you. You can carry them around with you and help yourself become calm in tense situations. Simply hold the stone of your choice on the fingers and allow your energy to flow. You'll notice your breathing patterns changing and inner sense of peace occurring. If you are in an extreme state of anxiety, you can use your crystals to rebalance your Chakras. Simply take the Quartz, place it at the center of your Solar Plexus Chakra and rotate the crystal slowly in a clockwise direction while breathing deeply. A few minutes later you should feel fine.

CHAPTER 10

Letting Go With Teragram ^{Sm} Therapy

The Power Of The Teragram

Finally, it is time to focus on Teragram^{sm} Therapy. This therapy is done with six colored Agate slices cut from geodes that are approximately two to three inches in diameter. Mini-Teragrams, which are about one inch in diameter, are also available and are equally as effective. Each Teragram, primarily Agate, has Quartz crystal within it. Any geode, when cut open, will reveal circles within it, just as a tree, when felled, will reveal the rings of its seasons. The secret of the power of the Teragram lies in the way the geode is formed. Energy passing through a Teragram must follow the natural circles of the Agate. The combination of Agate and Quartz creates a calm but forceful energy that will regenerate the energy flow of each major and minor Chakra in the body.

What Is A Chakra?

A Chakra is a major vortex of energy created by many minor vortices within. It can look like a hurricane, with swirling masses of color. If you could look into this miniature hurricane, you would see many tiny tornadoes whirling around inside. As I explained earlier, each Chakra is cone shaped, being wide at the front and narrow at the rear. I should state here that there is another school of thought in which all Chakras are described as being made from two cones that meet at the spine, and that all Chakras pass through the body horizontally. My Spirit Guides informed me that this was incorrect.

During my years of research, my Spirit Guides showed me how each Chakra has been created in a baby as it grows in the womb. I learned how these Chakras develop once a child is formed. I saw, through their eyes, how each Chakra begins to function as the Spirit of the child-to-be bonds with its mother and spiritually absorbs all that she is emotionally. I saw, in my own children, how their Chakras were stimulated by my every thought, emotion and action. I learned how each child was stimulated to respond to outside forces as these Chakras rotated and interacted with the mothers' life, even before birth.

My Spirit Guides showed me how each Chakra was originally created by a spark of spiritual energy generated by the Spirit that was to incarnate. These tiny spiritual vortices of energy are the very life force that connects each Spirit to its Physical body. These spiritual vortices generate energy, which stimulate what will become the glands of the body to grow and function. By the time a child is born, all the Chakras are fully in harmony with the mother's total life experiences and are operating throughout all Five Bodies. Every child is born with the gift of knowledge. Unfortunately, no one remembers!

Every vortex within every Chakra sends energy in a spiral clockwise direction from the front of the body to the back. At the back, energy is then forced to return to the front of the body in another clockwise spiral rotation. These overlapping spiral energies form a double helix. This double helix carries the DNA strand coded into every cell together with ancestral conditioning, the mother's history and the history of the child's spiritual experiences in past lives. All these vortices rotate at different speeds, rather like an old fashioned clock where different sized cogs rotate at different speeds to give the correct time. So each vortex within each Chakra rotates to give the right energy force that will provide an individual with balanced health and well-being.

Your Chakras Are Exactly Where They Should Be.

The Crown Chakra flows downward through the center of the body while the Base (Root) Chakra flows upward to cross over the Crown Chakra. The Heart and Solar Plexus Chakras are at the center where these two cones cross one another. This forms a diamond in the center of the body. Crossing diagonally through the body from right front to left rear is the Spleen Chakra, which ensures that each Spirit stays within the Physical Body. The Spleen Chakra is a most important Chakra. If it fails, a person will die. All these Chakras are interactive and constantly rotating and vibrating, spinning out energy that creates the Aura and directing flow within the Five Bodies. The rate of speed of the rotation of the Crown Chakra and Base (Root) Chakra controls the rate of the other five Chakras. If a person is negative, the rate slows.

Within each Chakra are the vortices that constantly struggle to harmonize and control the flow of energy in each body. Teragram^{sm} Therapy helps those vortices rotate at the right vibration, giving them maximum performance, which results in a more harmonious outlook on life.

Where To Use Teragrams

Teragram^{sm} Therapy may be used either on the front or rear of the body. If they are placed on the front of the Chakra, then physical and emotional balance will occur, followed by a spiritual awakening. If they are placed on the rear, Spiritual awareness in psychic development occurs rapidly, followed by an emotional and mental sense of well-being.

Teragrams may also be placed on parts of the body that are in pain or discomfort. Here, they will stimulate the Acu points, which in turn will allow energy to enter the meridian, causing a release of old issues from past memories through the Chakras.

Chakras Are Busy Bees

Each Chakra has a primary function, but is capable of integrating the other Chakras' vibrations within it. The Base (Root) Chakra is by its very nature, the densest. This is where all our unlearned lessons are stored waiting for us to repeat patterns that will stimulate this Chakra to release energy by spinning faster. When this occurs, our cellular-neuro-muscular memory is stimulated. Our ensuing actions stimulate us to try to understand others and ourselves a little better, in the spiritual hope that we will awaken to inner truths.

As we interact with others, we exchange with them. By desire, we send spiral energy from the Solar Plexus Chakra to another person. That person in turn does the same. In this way, we exchange energy. As we accept another person's energy into the Solar Plexus, it mixes with our own energy.

That energy then flows through the meridians to the Heart Chakra. There it is assimilated and subsequent emotions arise. Our emotional reaction opens the Heart Chakra, which allows us to send spiral energy to the other person. They do Likewise.

This new exchange of energy is integrated in this Chakra and then it is passed on to the Throat Chakra. We are naturally very vocal when talking about likes, dislikes and ourselves. As communication deepens, the Throat Chakra sends out spiral energy to the other person, who does likewise. This energy is then assimilated into the Throat Chakra.

Then this energy is moved on up to the Third Eye Chakra, where perceptions may be altered by the introduction of this new energy. Here ideas about self and the other person become alive with hopes and dreams.

Now these two Chakras exchange energies, which stimulate the Crown Chakra to conclude the joining of two people and the subsequent awareness about themselves that has arisen. The brain assimilates all this information, creating more energy, which is then passed back down through the Chakras to the Spleen Chakra where the Five Bodies are balanced and harmonized.

When the conversation with another is inspiring and stimulating, the two people involved will develop a bond, which may lead to permanent friendship. If the conversation is negative, these two people would still be exchanging energies, creating a negative bond, drawn from a need to know more about themselves and their fears. In the overview, any interaction is a good one, because it allows each one to know more about him/herself, by interfacing with others. In the spiritual sense, if you really know yourself, then you also know everyone else.

There Is More To Physical Union Than You Know!

In a sexual relationship, the Base Chakra is stimulated by sexual activities. During orgasm, energy flows up the spine through each of the Chakras where it forces an exchange of energy through the front of each Chakra. Most feel the Base, Solar Plexus and Heart Chakras spinning with wild sensations when an orgasm occurs. It also interacts with the Throat Chakra, stimulating words of wonder and pleasure. Few realize how active the Third Eye and Crown Chakras are at this time. At that moment, there is a shift is the sense of self and an awakening of a truth. Most couples are full of fear and subliminally refuse to see or listen to this part. They are lost in the pleasure and the comfort of their partner.

Often the Spleen Chakra is busy trying to find a new balance in the energy flow of the Five Bodies. Tantric yoga teaches the art of controlling and sensing all the Chakras at the moment of orgasm. If the connection is made among all the Chakras, the energy will flow all the way to the Crown, where a firework display of energy can be seen in geometric forms. The Spleen Chakra balances the remaining energy, which leads that individual into a new level of material and spiritual awareness.

Well Mend It, Dear One, Mend It!

If a Chakra is weak and in need of rebalancing, then Teagram[sm] Therapy is the easiest and quickest way to do it. It can even be done watching TV. All that you see, hear, touch, taste and smell are stimuli that cause your Chakras to rotate. If you are full of fear, anxiety, worries, and negative emotions, then your Chakras will need some work. You can change your energies by watching or becoming involved with activities while wearing a Teragram or two. Place one Teragram each on the Solar Plexus and Heart Chakras. You will find that your attitude and energy levels will have changed by the end of the day. You will be calmer and more able to cope with your problems.

The way it works is simple. When your five senses focus on something, your conscious mind searches for any similar things in your past. It finds many events, which are then assimilated into one focus. This results in a conscious awareness and subsequent emotions arise. Then you make a decision to become afraid or angry, etc. At that point, you are negatively gripped by your past, and can feel yourself choking on it. Wearing or sitting with a Teragram will help dissipate the negative memories and tone down or erase the emotions. It will help you make your assessment of your situation and the thing you focused on to fit into a more sensible form that makes it possible for you to manage comfortably.

Several years ago, an old client came to visit me. At that time, I was still experimenting with the Teragrams. I had just placed Teragrams on her Heart and Solar Plexus Chakras when the telephone rang. It was a distress call. Someone wanted to kill herself. I left my client visitor watching "Shark Week" on The Discovery Channel. I was over an hour helping my client on the phone. When I returned to my visitor, she greeted me with, "What were you doing to me. I was watching those sharks. I hate sharks! They frighten the life out of me. Anyway, I was watching those sharks, when I felt energy moving around my body. I felt you healing me."

I informed her that I had done nothing. I had almost forgotten she was still in my house while dealing with the client on the telephone. I explained how the Teragrams work, and how they neutralize negative emotions. When she thought about what I was saying, she let me know that she then realized that she was no longer afraid of sharks. "They're just big fish," she said and laughed.

So, watch a horror film, and watch your worst nightmares disappear. Listen to emotional, sentimental stories, and find your own emotions balancing. Teragram℠ Therapy is, in my opinion, one of the best ways to help myself. I never go anywhere without them.

If you want to feel more dedicated to yourself, try lying down and placing a Teragram on all the Chakras from the Third Eye on down. Each Chakra has an essential color, so it helps to build them up, if you use the right one.

The colors are listed below. Lie down and place Teragrams on yourself:
- Third Eye Chakra Violet
- Throat Chakra Blue
- Heart Chakra Green
- Solar Plexus Chakra Pink

- Base (Root) Chakra Red

Sit up and hold Teragrams:
- Spleen Chakra Red and Blue
- Crown Chakra Natural

The Spleen Chakra is best balanced while sitting up. One Teragram should be held in each hand. The Left hand should hold the *blue* one. Place the left hand holding the Teragram flat to the rear left, over the spleen, while holding the *red* Teragram over the front right side, over the liver. Allow yourself to feel your energy flowing back and forth through the Teragrams. Think "Balance." Visualize some scales with numbers 0 –100. Push the indicator to 50. Then you know you are balanced.

For the Crown Chakra, place the *natural* Teragram on the top center point of your head. Place the palm of the left hand over it. Then place the palm of the right hand on top of the left. Take deep breaths and visualize golden light. You will feel yourself becoming lighter and more relaxed. You will intuitively know when you have done it long enough. During this focus, you may experience sensations in and around your body, as well as extra-sensory perception. You may even contact your Spirit Guides.

On other occasions, you may wish to vary the colors. It is okay to place Teragrams according to your intuition. Your first spontaneous choice is the right one. Each Chakra can need color for different parts of its rotation. You may need a certain color healing on the Etheric Body in one Chakra, while another may need the same color in the Spirit Body. So exchange Teragrams and trust yourself that you have chosen the right colors for each Chakra. There is no damage done if you should select one that is not needed. All that happens is that the Chakra you have placed it on will make no changes.

You Can Help Others Too

If you are the therapist, then the Teragrams can be placed on your client/patient who is then left alone for a short period. You can then return and change them around and leave them for another period of time. This of course, can be done several times in one half-hour session.

Each Teragram is capable of absorbing your healing energy, and amplifying it, as your energy passes through it. This will help you to rebuild your own/client/patient's Chakras. By placing your healing fingers gently on the Teragram, or placing your Palm Chakra over the Teragram, you will be able to feel electrical impulses that show a return of energy when the Chakra is rebuilt. If the Chakra is overloaded, you will have a sensation of resistance, together with a vibration that is felt as an electrical charge causing your hand to tremble in a refined shake.

If the Chakra is in need of healing in the *Subtle Bodies*, then your hand should be held about four inches away from the Chakra. Your hand should be extended and held flat with the palm facing the body. Your hand should then begin a clockwise rotation as though polishing a fine piece of furniture. Hand rotation at this height over the Teragram will cause a change in the Etheric Body.

For a similar effect on the Spirit Body, hold your hand about twelve inches away from the Physical Body and do the same movement over the Teragram. Rotating the hands over the Teragrams can also affect the Higher Mind and Soul Bodies. Hold your hand at a further distance from the body. Use your intuition and feel. Then rotate. Notice any physical reactions in yourself/patient/client. There will be some ideo-motor responses, though possibly very slight.

If you or client/patient have back problems, then lie or have them lie on their front and put the Teragrams on the rear Chakras. Do exactly the same as you would for the front. Your healing connection will be more directly in tune with the Spirit, Higher Mind and Soul Bodies of yourself/ patient/client. People with back problems are individuals who have a fear of their own spiritual power and are unable to trust themselves. On a conscious level, they are always trying to control someone or something. Teragram[sm] Therapy on these people works wonders for them.

Dust The Cobwebs Away!

On occasion, it may be necessary to dust the cobwebs from the Aura. As we go about our daily business, we pass equipment, computers, animals, other people, and so on. We pick up many different sensations that never reach our conscious mind. Those mixed up energies are not necessarily an integral part of learning, but rather more of what has been learned. Those things that we are used to and have mastered do have an effect on us, in that they tend to stay with us and clog us up. Like the saying, "A new broom sweeps clean," so, the Aura needs a clean out.

To cleanse the Aura, take any Teragram of your choice. Hold it with the tips of the fingers so the Teragram is exposed. Now make sweeping movements up and down, in and out, round and about in circular and diagonal sweeps as though painting the Aura. Do this all around yourself/patient/client's body, and above the head. To cleanse the outer perimeter, extend your movements outward to approximately three or four feet away from the physical form. Have someone do your Aura for you. Remember that each body has its own vibration, which extends way beyond the human form. When you have finished, dowse the Aura with your hands to find its perimeter. You will find there is a definite resistance to your hand entering the surface of the outer field of the Aura. When you feel this, you will know that the client is well protected.

Relax In Meditation.

If you are of a mind to meditate, Teragrams are an excellent tool to use. Place them over the Chakras and trust yourself to let go. Relax. Take deep breaths. Feel the Teragrams working. Then visualize the colors of the rainbow. As you do this, your thoughts transform the color into a vibration. This change in vibration will affect the Chakras. Watch how you interpret these changes. Now visualize silver, copper, gold, lilac, and watch as these thoughts create higher vibrations within you.

Your Teragrams will help you stabilize any fear you may have about connecting with the Spirit World and any subsequent changes that may occur. Next, think of electric blue, which is the color of the Holy Spirit. This thought will allow you to lift your energy and harmonize with Spirit. Your Teragrams will help you balance. Then enjoy!

Let's Get Things Straight!

As a result of many of my clients' requests, I have made an audiocassette and CD with two meditations to help individuals become aware of the effective use of Teragrams. One of the meditations deals with the alignment of the Five Bodies. Aligning the Five Bodies is a must. Imagine driving your car with unbalanced wheels. You would soon wear out the tires and have a blowout, on top of having a noisy and bumpy ride. If your Five Bodies are out of alignment, then it can be equally uncomfortable for you. You may feel out of sorts, as though something is not quite right with you. You may have weird sensations that make you fearful for no apparent reason. Your emotions may be affected in that you are unstable and irrational. Psychic phenomena, making you panic, may be happening. Unusual body sensations may send you cringing as you feel the imbalance of the Five Bodies. It is very important to put the Teragrams on each Chakra immediately while lying down and to visualize the Five Bodies harmonizing. Pictorial visualization will bring the bodies into line. The following is one of the many methods that I have found to work efficiently:

Visualize yourself standing in front of a mirror. As you look, you recognize your Soul Body that is filled with golden light. As you look, you become a golden light. Take a deep breath and feel this movement in your physical form. Now visualize the mirror again and see yourself. As you look, recognize your Higher Mind Body and see yourself becoming an electric blue color. Become the color all over, and feel yourself changing. Now visualize the mirror again and see yourself. As you look, recognize your Spirit Body. It is yellow all over and as you see yourself turn yellow, you feel it flowing all over your Physical Body. Feel yourself changing. Now again, visualize yourself in the mirror. As you look, you see yourself becoming green all over. Now recognize your Etheric Body and sense the changes occurring in your Physical Body. Now visualize yourself in the mirror and see all the colors of the rainbow blending. You become white light. All your bodies are now aligned. Your Teragrams have helped you to harmonize and balance the Five Bodies with the Chakras. Now it is important to close the Chakras.

Claim Your Own Space!

Closing the Chakras simply means creating a vibration that causes them to rotate at a slightly faster rate than when open and sharing yourself. This act of closing simply reminds you to keep your energy to yourself. We are by nature and through spiritual desire, open and receptive to one another. Therefore, we readily open our energies up to others and, in so doing, give some of our energy away. In response, someone will give us energy back. We exchange ourselves this way.. Closing the Chakras simply means giving an order to refrain from sharing yourself with anyone. When the Chakras are closed, they rotate faster, creating a resistant whirl, which, like a wind, blows people away. Those who are closed are left alone. Under the Law of Karma, "No one fragment may impose its will on another at any time on any level". So, by closing your Chakras, people must leave you alone.

Your Spirit Knows Best!

The Crown Chakra is the exception. It remains open to the higher vibrations. You are constantly in touch with God and your Spirit Guides through this Chakra. You are also in touch with everyone else through the sensations that you receive from other people's auras. It is this Chakra that tells you to open or close. Through your brain impulses, you receive a mental picture and make a choice. This is a spontaneous thing that happens. It is part of the survival package brought by your Spirit into the body.

Close the Chakras by visualizing each one and physically pulling the muscles in over the areas of the Chakras and saying, "Close." With practice, this can be done in one spasm wave from head to tail, including the Chakras in the elbows, hands, knees and feet. It should be noted that the elbow and knee Chakras are rarely opened. Negativity creates a need to fight, so these two Minor Chakras do not open until an individual has evolved away from fear and is able to totally enjoy life. Usually, these Minor Chakras open in the later years. However, It is always a good idea to check them. See my book, *50 Spiritually Powerful Meditations*, for directed meditations to close down all the chakras.

People who have painful elbows need to create their own space. Usually, they are too busy trying to fight their way through the maddening crowd. Those who have painful knees are usually too conceited and controlling. They need a general lesson in humility and tolerance. No matter what your problem, use of Teragram^{sm} Therapy will help. It is non-invasive and very compatible with any other medical treatments or therapies.

CHAPTER 11

The Nature Of Your Spirit Body

I Think, Therefore I Am

Throughout this book, I have mentioned the different ways the mind affects the Five Bodies. It is possible for each of us to see and believe what we see. Our imagination can create believable scenarios for meditation and we allow ourselves to trust in them. We can visualize something negative and we can immediately believe it is true. We can conjure up a visual monster and scare ourselves to death. In reverse, we can see things and reject them as stupid and not worthy of a second look. In one single moment we can make up our mind that what we saw was just imagination and nothing worthy of remembrance.

So what is it that constantly makes us shift our pictures around? What is it that drives us to try to understand the way we think? Why is it we remember something we did when we were ten, and cannot remember what we did last week? Why do we have so many ideas about everything and think we know all, when really we hardly understand a thing?

Well, try this answer: It is your Spirit that is constantly trying new ways to find itself. Your Spirit has flitted from life to life like a butterfly. Time after time, it is drawn to the strange and unusual. It constantly seeks a challenge, an opportunity to grow, and it will do it by any means. Earth is a wonderful playground for your Spirit to explore many avenues. Here you can be an actor and take on many roles in varying ways in which it will challenge you to look deeper inside and question yourself. It doesn't matter who you were, or what you will be in the next life. It only matters that you enjoy this one.

Role-Playing Can Be Fun!

So, how can you enjoy this life when it is filled with all kinds of negativity? How can you possibly have fun being an actor when no one lets you play? Well, that's the craft that you must develop. You must try to find a way that makes you noticed and accepted. You'll do anything to get that praise and support. You'll nag, scream, and shout if the role calls for it. Alternatively, maybe you'll sing sweet songs and praise others, so they notice you. You have to work hard at it. You need to train yourself to think ahead. Don't program it, but be prepared for the worst! Every little thing you do might not be noticed and you can't have that. Therefore, you have to do it with fanfare and class. The bigger the better! Perhaps you're over-doing it? Maybe you should play it down a touch! Pretend you're not so important so that others will see how poor and downtrodden you are. That might be nice! A little rest while you let others wait on you and bug you every time you don't pull your weight. Such a dilemma! So many choices to make and so many ways to do it. Small wonder that your Spirit is depressed. Or is it?

Actually, your Spirit is having a whale of a time. In fact, sometimes it is so busy, lost in the role, that it forgets why it is here on this Earth. The truth is, your Spirit needs to find a clue to its existence. It has been searching so long for something that it's almost forgotten what it is. But, deep inside, every so often, it remembers. It remembers it must find its way to the collective consciousness that is the Universal Mind of God and embrace unconditional love. It must become one with God.

So why does your Spirit get stuck in a rut? Well, the truth is it's scared of the unknown. Scared of being God. Afraid of losing its identity and the opportunity of being anything it wants to be. It's hard enough being the boss at work! How could one possibly be boss over everything? Of course, being God is not quite the same, but in the long run, the basic emotion is the same. One must have a love of oneself and be able to function to the best of one's ability. One must be creative.

So, now that you have taken a look at your Spirit, it is time to see the role you have taken on. You've copied everyone you've met and integrated yourself very well. Do you like the way you set yourself up? Do you think you could do with a few changes here and there? Maybe you think that things are not good enough? Well, now is the time to change. Be creative and develop a new role. Find one that has more character, more charisma and more action. Perhaps a new career would be in order or a different kind of social life. Even a few new family members and friends might change things.

Your Spirit can create all these ideas and more. Your brain is capable of collecting data and re-arranging it to suit the role. With a little shift here and there in your Five Bodies, you could pull it off if you want to. Do you want to? Of course, that is the big question. Why should you change after all the hard work you've put out from the beginning in creating the role you have. Maybe the role you have is fine, but you just have not figured out how to make the best of it. Perhaps you need an advisor, a Guardian Angel or two to help you redesign yourself. Naturally, they are there when you need them. The only problem is, you've got so lost in the role, and you've forgotten how to connect to them. So, maybe it is best to dump the role after all?

Okay, so you decide to change roles, but what if all those people you've met and conditioned to accept you as you are, won't know you any more? They'll think you are someone else. So what if you lose them! Many of them never connected to you in the first place. However, there are those few you did connect with. What about them? It's a chance you have to take. Maybe they will still recognize you after the change.

Of course, your Spirit is scared. It wants to be remembered by everyone. It wants to belong to everyone. Unfortunately, not everyone wants to belong to it. Well, those Soul Fears sure do keep rearing their ugly heads. So the battle continues. I need to be alone to change, but I want people to watch and approve the change. I want to be successful, but I want people to critique me, to prevent me from losing the role. I want unconditional love to ooze out from everyone I encounter and most important of all, I want to be able to love everyone unconditionally myself.

You Are A Priceless Treasure.

Do you think your Spirit is worth the time and effort? I do. Without its own truth, there is no Spirit. Without its need to survive, there is no life. It is important to give your Spirit everything it needs to make the role work that you've created here on Earth. It needs you to get that mind into ship-shape working order. Those emotions need to be cleaned up and balanced. The good ones can heal the bad ones. And, that body! It probably needs an overhaul. You need lots of activities to help it get fit and plenty of interactions that will allow your Spirit to walk tall in the physical body.

Now you're beginning to get the idea! Make a date to plan your future. Work with your Crystal Acupuncture^sm and Teragram^sm Therapies to create a new role, or improve the old one. Spend lots of time in balanced contemplation. Meditate, and awaken to your connections with your Spirit Guides. Enjoy yourself with fun activities, good friends and happy occasions. Share your feelings and appreciate everything you've created. Pat yourself on the back and say "Well done. I've got a good life." Moreover, all those negative people you worried about, well they're all leaving, looking for a new role themselves. So, they won't be bothering you any more.

Love Is 'A Many Splendored Thing!' Or Is It?

Wow! Emotions are running high and life is scary with all these new things to see and do. Trying to understand all these new emotions can be very hard at times. Emotions can be so strong! Sometimes they run away with you. You can lose yourself in negative emotions. It's a good role to play for a while as you find out who your true friends are. But even they get fed up watching you play this role. Of course, there are other emotions like anger and fear. You could try playing ball with anger. Toss it back and forth, and see who drops the ball first. Then you can blame them for ruining the game. Perhaps it might be better to have a contest and find out who is the real coward.

Whatever role you take, negative emotions can be fun for a while, until you get stuck in them. Then you find yourself trying to escape, but the more you move, the more stuck you become. Rather like falling into a big vat of chewing gum on a hot sunny day. There's no getting that stuff off, unless, of course, you do something radical like using a chemical. Then you come out squeaky clean and bare. Bare is nice, but bare is clean and empty. No emotions! Nothing but numbness! It seems safe to sit on the fence and wait for something to happen. You can sit awhile until you are thoroughly bored. Then what? A strange emotion arises out of the depth of your inner self. Passion! Such desire for something – anything — to happen, and it does. Why, before you know it you're off that fence and back in the game. And, amazingly, you've entered a new role; one that seems to make you happy. You laugh and sing a lot, and often demonstrate your creative self. You feel deeply, and your mind is enjoying itself digesting all this new information. Your Spirit? Well, it's back on track enjoying a new experience and loving every minute of it. Happiness abounds. No secrets, no fears, no anger or shame. No judgment or blame. Only joy and bliss! WOW! It's love!

Change Is As Good As A Rest!

So, whatever happened to that fear of change? Somewhere along the line, it turned into a challenge with excellent opportunities to gain more. Yes, *greed*, that so-called ugly sin, reared its head and pulled you on. Those things you needed. Those people you wanted. They were the sprats to catch a bigger fish, the mackerel. You took the hook and got pulled into a new direction before you even knew it. So, once the change was made, there was nothing left to do but develop it. Good Luck!

Of course, you don't really need luck, just a good attitude and a lot of will power to promote yourself in this new role. Throw a party. Make new friends. Embrace new philosophies and find a cause that suits your taste. Action speaks louder than words. Everyone will notice you and like you, even love you.

Confidence comes with positive affirmations and good responses. Build up your self-esteem, worth and value. Think well of yourself in all aspects. Appreciate your talents and the skills you have used in creating this role, and let others appreciate you too. All this effort in becoming the person you are must be worth a whole bunch. In addition, all that time and energy you spend in doing things must have some value in your life. Better not waste it! Isn't it time to fly high and touch the sky?

CHAPTER 12

Reprogramming Cellular Memory

I Remember It Well! We Tell Ourselves Too Much.

Reprogramming the cellular-neuro-muscular memory is as easy as falling off a bicycle. There was a time in my early teens when I first learned to ride a bicycle around London, England. I had very little road experience and was very nervous. On two occasions, I borrowed a friend's bicycle and rode several miles around the city and local parks. I was thrilled to feel the wind in my hair. Though nothing harmful happened, I was constantly on the lookout for danger.

By the time, I had completed the second ride; I was beginning to feel terrified of the traffic and the journey to the park. A last attempt came a few weeks later when I borrowed the bicycle again. This time, I actually fell off and lay on the ground in an emotional panic. Of course, I picked myself up, dusted myself down, and rode home. I had no choice. I had to get the bicycle back to its owner. Along that journey, I told myself how stupid I was to be afraid. By the time I arrived home, I had convinced myself that I was a good rider. I felt I had successfully conquered this skill.

Years later, my sons tried to get me to ride their bikes. I lovingly refused, announcing that I was too old for that sort of thing. At that moment, I realized just how afraid I was and covered it up with excuses. I never did ride their bikes.

In my forties, I found the courage to ride again. My fear was still apparent. I was dreadfully afraid of falling and breaking my bones. Nevertheless, I pressed myself to ride regularly, justifying it as a needed exercise. Each time I rode the bike, I reminded myself of the fall I had had as a teenager. Those constant thoughts kept my fear alive. Finally, one day, my worst fear happened. I was riding to a halt at a traffic light, when I lost my balance. As I fell, I found myself observing myself in slow motion. In those microseconds, I reminded myself how to fall, and to protect my head as well as to enjoy the experience. I heard two women exclaiming their fear for me in various forms of "oohs" and "ahs", which sounded strange and yet funny. By the time I landed, I was in a fit of giggles with the bike on top of me. My emotions were sharp as fear left me and was replaced with a rational sense of safety and a full picture of myself sprawled in the gutter. In that moment I reprogrammed myself and now ride without fear of falling.

The point of this story is to show how our senses are heightened during moments of fear and anxiety. These negative emotions cause us to immediately move into a state of hypnosis. During that time, we are telling ourselves to accept these fears and the evidence that supports the fear. We make a belief and stick to it. My second fall was a positive one. Instead of being afraid, I was laughing. During that time, my fearful emotions still took me into a state of hypnosis as I fell, but the pictorial images that I created, together with my awareness of self preservation and humor helped me to hypnotize myself into deleting the old idea and replacing it with a new one.

The Pictures Stuck In My Mind!

Emotions are the glue that helps us retain our memories. Every action we take, whether it is stretching, running, falling, or simply sitting calls for an emotion to stimulate the body to move. That emotion may be negative or positive. Whatever we desire simulates us to try to get it. If we fail to achieve our goal, we become emotionally negative. Body movement, however slight, is associated with emotions all the time. Happy events are also encoded into the Physical Body.

Unfortunately, we focus more on the negative events. Your mind can associate throwing a ball with reaching into the cupboard. Raising the arm stimulates the brain to remember all the many other times you have raised it. During that time, your sub-conscious is recalling all the emotional details. Those emotional details are recreated in pictorial form. Then you've got the picture in your conscious mind, along with an emotion that seems to control your every move. Old aches and pains manifest out of nowhere. You feel out of sorts and emotionally low. Of course, the reverse can happen too!

When your body begins to break down, it is telling you to stop what you are doing and to remember things that were similar in the past. It is then that you must meditate and release the old memories along with the emotions that made it stick. If you can't meditate, then find a Hypnotherapist who can help you into a hypnotic state. Then you can pull up all your associated memories and deprogram them by simply allowing the emotion that has manifested to be released. Once the emotion is seen to be an obstacle, the conscious mind can easily adapt by pulling on another emotion to erase the first.

It works this way. Think of a really sad time. Pull that memory right into the front of your mind and wallow in the emotions. Now think of a really good time and remember the emotions. Notice how the negative emotion has disappeared. It is impossible for both emotions to be felt at once. If one tries to feel them both at the same time, then neutrality is the result. It is very possible for the mind to be indifferent to situations in your past. It is just a question of reshuffling your thoughts.

Another way to change your negative emotions is to pictorially pull up a memory. Look first at the serious pictures you recall. Then study the emotional effect those feelings have on you and your body. Now take that picture and change it. Turn it into a cartoon. For example: You have a memory of being slapped across the face by your girlfriend. You feel mentally destroyed and emotionally heart-broken. Now you recreate the scene. Your girl friend is standing on the edge of a precipice. She is about to fall when she reaches out in desperation and slaps you.

As she totters on the edge, you see the cartoon effect. Her hands are waving frantically around as she tries to save herself from her "ginormous" skirt, which is wrapped around her face. She looks funny as her body twists and turns.

You reach out to try to catch her, but you are laughing too much. You watch her falling, with her skirt catching the wind. She drifts away like a balloon and you know she is safe and that you are okay. These pictorial images will be retained in the subconscious. Whenever you try to think of the serious side of this relationship, you will automatically think of the cartoon you have made. In no time at all, you will overcome the negative memories.

Relive The Drama One More Time!

Lying or sitting in a comfortable position where you can use your crystals to do Crystal Acupuncture^{sm} and Teragram^{sm} Therapies at the same time is invaluable when trying to erase negative history. First, place the Teragrams on the Throat, Heart, Solar Plexus and Base (Root) Chakras and then stimulate the five meridians from your fingertips with a Quartz crystal. As you stimulate (impound) the meridians, think of your life and select an old memory that has given you pain over the years. Continue to stimulate the points. Watch, as the memory becomes clearer and the emotions stronger. Let yourself truly relive the feeling. Watch as your Chakras rebalance repeatedly. Let all your emotional associations with this memory also arise. That is allowing the drama to unfold. Do not analyze the thoughts that arise, but rather observe them.

When you feel you have sufficiently stimulated the memory, select an Amethyst crystal and simply hold it on the fingertip Meridian points and allow your energies to flow. You will feel a release in the body. Your mind will begin to accept that changes are in order, as you energize your Spirit Body. Inspirational awareness will manifest and as it does, a good thought will send a positive emotion to the surface. Now rotate this Amethyst crystal on the points and watch as the positive emotion takes hold. Now tell yourself you have a new positive feeling. The more you feel the positive emotions, the better you become.

Put Your Self In A Bind

Sometimes it works better to tell oneself opposing things. For example, tell yourself that the more negative you feel, the more positive you become. This is called a double bind. Your mind has to make a choice. It hates a dilemma and will more than likely select the positive one. Work on yourself for about one hour and then close the Chakras.

Mixing Therapies Can Do A Person A World Of Good

It may be that you are the therapist and wish to work with Aromatherapy and Reflexology along with Crystal Acupuncture^sm and Teragram^sm Therapy. Begin by placing the Teragrams on the Chakras. Then apply Aromatherapy oils to the neck and feet of your client/patient to stimulate the neural senses. Then begin with a Reflexology treatment to the feet, which will stimulate the meridians to open. When you have finished both feet, use Crystal Acupuncture^sm on the tip of each of the five toes to complete the treatment. If necessary rebuild the Chakras, then tone and balance and close them after treatment.

If a full massage is given, the Teragrams can still be placed either on the front or back of your client/patient. If working a Chakra area, the Teragram should be removed. Replace it after massage is completed in this area. Energy will flow through the Teragram again. You may choose to put your hand on the Teragram during massage to help balance the Chakra. However, you may wish to leave that until the massage is finished. This is entirely up to you and your state of awareness as you focus on what your client/patient needs.

Dowsing For The Right Crystal.

If knots and painful areas are found during the massage, Crystal Acupuncture^sm can be used. Simply dowse the area with your hand. Try to sense the shape of the Aura by holding the hand approximately four feet away from the client's body. Slowly bring the hand towards the client, feeling for a weakness in the Aura. Your intuitive self will feel which body carries the weakness. If your hand senses lack of resistance in the outer area of the Aura, then a Quartz crystal should be used to stimulate the nearest meridian point beneath your hand. This client will have bad energy flow in all the bodies. Dowse the body, looking for levels of resistance. Select crystals according to the distance your hand ends up from the physical body. Remember, the closer you are to the physical form, the more you have to work on the Physical Body.

If the problem is in the Etheric Body, then your hand will have no resistance about four to six inches from the Physical Body. If the Spirit Body is unbalanced, then your hand will cease to feel resistance about twelve inches from the Physical Body. Should your hand find no resistance in the Higher Mind Body, then you must select Hematite or Sodalite to stimulate energy in the Physical body, making it receptive to the Subtle Bodies. A person who has a problem in the Subtle Bodies is usually mentally disturbed, in shock, in a coma, or paralyzed in fear.

If this is the case, regular Crystal Acupuncture[sm] Treatments with Teragram[sm] Therapy should be given at least three times a week. Remember, the Aura can be brushed and fluffed with Teragrams to release the 'cobwebs" of their mind along with the emotional trauma that originally caused the client to become ill. Most illnesses are not in the Physical Body. More often than not, they are in the Etheric Body. On rare occasions, the Spirit Body can be the cause.

Get Them Bones Connected

At various times, I have found my body seizing up on me. My shoulders have grown tense, which has caused my spine to misalign. Then my hips have dropped. By the time, I have taken full notice of what has happened to me, I find I am deeply troubled about my security. When I was a child, life was often threatening. My education about life included post-war traumas. I grew up clinging to everything I had, while constantly hoping for more. Each time I try to gain more support in a material sense, my Etheric Body gets out of sync with my Spirit Body, which causes my Physical Body to become misaligned.

First, I visit my chiropractor. As he moves my bones gently back into their correct position, I can feel my energies beginning to flow again. As soon as possible, I return home and meditate. I look at the things that I have been doing lately. I find the emotional cause and then work on myself to release that fear. To do this, I always use my Crystal Acupuncture[sm] techniques first and then the Teragrams while I am meditating.

Chiropractic work is extremely important. If my clients agree, I may realign them with shiatsu, deep muscular manipulation, and minor chiropractic movements after I have used Crystal Acupuncture^{sm} on the meridians to force open any blocks. When energy is flowing again, the bones return to their natural position very easily. It is possible to work on your own bones. Open up the blocks in your own body with Crystal Acupuncture^{sm} and then simply move yourself about with body twists, bends and stretches. Watch as everything pops back into place.

If you find you have a stubborn area, then meditate with the Teragrams on that area and bring an associated memory to the surface of your mind. Search for the emotion. Release it with deep breathing. Let energy flow through the stubborn area. Finish the meditation and exercise the body part while making a positive statement aloud. This statement must be directly opposing the negative emotion that had been stored in the stubborn area. For example, "I'm lonely," should be replaced with "I'm full of life."

Even The Impossible Is Possible.

Once in a while, I have dealt with healing malfunctions of the body caused by genetic deformity of the x-y factor in the way certain chromosomes divide. Nature seems to have played a wild hoax on those persons. But, despite this problem, I have helped individuals get around it by using Crystal Acupuncture^{sm} to stimulate other parts of the body, which will compensate as much as possible. One can never say that there is a cure, but one can say that there is an improvement.

I have worked with extremely autistic children and had excellent results. Paraplegics have found the use of their limbs again. Children with Leukemia have gone into remission. Cancer patients have had their lymphatic system and organs repaired. I could quote many scenarios, but whatever the case, the clients were able to trust themselves and the treatment. In some cases, the client was doubtful, but had faith in me. The rational mind can hinder repair, but it cannot fight the changes that occur in the energy flow of the Five Bodies. Negative thinking simply delays the healing process. Crystal Acupuncture^{sm} and Teragram^{sm} Therapies deal with subtle energies that the conscious mind cannot rationalize or explain. Therefore, the conscious mind has no defense against subtle change.

Over the years, I have had numerous occasions to use Crystal Acupuncture^{sm} on young babies and animals. These small clients had no awareness of what I was doing. This validates the assertion that the power of Crystal Acupuncture^{sm} as a healing tool is not controlled in anyway by a leap of faith and a conscious decision to believe in a cure from it. Children and animals are constantly in a state of surrender. This allows energy to be moved without resistance. A natural release leads to acceptance of the healing hand and an abundance of love that allows each body in the child or animal to harmonize. In the following chapter, you will read of several cases in which I have been responsible for helping individuals of all ages, as well as animals of all kinds to recover from illness.

CHAPTER 13

Case Studies

Doing The Right Thing!

A case involving a child with Tay Sachs Disease was one of the most interesting cases I had to deal with. Simply put, this is a disease caused by two people with low levels (50%) of the necessary enzymes in their brains, who created a child, who produced less than 50% or none at all. These enzymes break up the fatty acids that accumulate in the brain. If the brain does not rid itself of fatty acids, it eventually fails to function. All five senses eventually fail, and then the child begins to slowly die. A child born with this disease has no life expectancy beyond two years.

In this case, his Japanese mother, who had once been my interpreter, brought her little boy to me. Having worked closely with me, she knew about my therapies. I had never heard of this disease when she brought him to me. I taught her everything I knew about Crystal Acupuncture^{sm} and Teragram^{sm} Therapy and other therapies such as Aromatherapy and Reflexology. She then returned home.

Two weeks later, I flew to Japan. I was shocked when I saw him. He was a rag doll. His eyes said nobody was home. For one month, I lived with her, while I worked on him. Every day I stimulated his meridians, toned, and balanced his Chakras. Each night I worked the meridians in the brain, sectioning off the skull into 5mm squares. One by one, I worked those points. Daily, I gave him spinal Crystal Acupuncture℠ along with physiotherapy. By the time I was ready to leave, there was only one thing left to do. I took him to the nearest temple, blessed him and placed him in God's hands.

The changes in this little boy were enormous. His eyes were alert. He watched people cross the room. He held his head up and sometimes kicked and flailed his legs and arms. Both his mother and I knew that he would never be normal, but at least he now had some sense of his existence. He was smiling and definitely reacting with all his five senses. His mother lovingly continued to give him his treatments and to get medical support and regular physiotherapy for him.

She moved back to America and his treatments continued. The last time I saw him he was turning four years old, and was doing as well as could be expected for a child with such a terrible disease. My therapies had helped him to live much longer than anyone had ever expected.

A friend of mine, a dedicated minister, suddenly had a stroke. I immediately rushed to her side. She was facing the ordeal of being paralyzed down the left side of her body. I stimulated, toned and balanced all her meridians, giving particular attention to the meridians that worked the brain in the area of the stroke. Then, I rebuilt all her Chakras with the use of Teragram℠ Therapy. By this time, she was in a state of hypnosis. I took her deeper and told her to sense the Teragrams and their power. She could feel them well. I then told her that all her energies were returning to their normal flow and that her body would repair.

Daily, she would grow stronger and find full use of her body once more. I told her that the Teragrams were her friends, and that she would use them every day to meditate with them, as she made herself better. She is now fully recovered and still speaking of how she made herself better all by herself. The combination of Crystal Acupuncture℠ with Teragram℠ Therapy and hypnosis is a powerful tool when healing someone.

A young boy of seventeen broke his back in a motorbike accident. His sister was one of my students and an excellent healer. She and her boyfriend, another of my students, visited him daily. I visited him each night through astral travel. For one year, the boy was in hospital and for one year, I visited him each night. No one told him about me. When he was released from the hospital, everyone was excited. This was the time to find out if all the healing his sister and boyfriend had given him with their crystals had worked.

On the day in question, I arrived to put him into hypnosis and check him out. He went in easily. The first thing I asked him was if he knew who I was. His response was. "Yes, you're the lady who came and sat on my bed every night and told me I would walk again." This was clear evidence that he had accepted me on a spiritual level, although his conscious mind had no idea who I was. I then took him deeper into hypnosis. He was asked to go back in his mind to the earlier hours of the day of the accident. I told him that he would physically relive the accident without the trauma. He was instructed to allow his mind to observe this time without fear.

He described how he was on the motorbike. He described the scenes along the road. He felt good. Then he saw the events leading up to the accident. He swore and then curled his body up into a ball. We knew then that his physical body was healed. I then told him to relax and that all memory of the fear of that accident was gone. I told him that when he awakened he would remember that he had curled himself up into a ball and that he would find that he could now move as his mind instructed him to though spontaneous impulses. He was then awakened.

Before the session, he had been strapped into his seat. He was now able to hold himself upright. He could move both legs. It appeared a miracle had happened. He was taken to the hospital for physiotherapy. He began to tone his muscles. I left him in the care of his mother and sister and went to live in America. As this young man began to recover, his emotions took over. He knew that if he got better, he would not have the attention he had been getting. Slowly, those emotions took over, and slowly he retreated into himself. He refused to do his therapy and once again became muscle bound. Unfortunately, he has a body that is healed, but a mind that is not.

Here is an example of a child needing love so badly, that he will sacrifice his body to get it. Ten years later, I tried to hypnotize him again. He resisted, so I knew it was impossible to help him. He wanted to be paralyzed. In fact, I could see that all his muscles had atrophied and the ligaments had tightened, making it impossible to move the joints. What a shame! The power of the mind can be very destructive when negative emotions control all thoughts.

A lady had many emotional problems in her life. Her husband had been unfaithful to her. She had troubles with her children. Each child had a problem with her. She could not see that she was a problem to her husband either. She brought each member of the family to me in the hope that I would change them and make them the way she wanted them to be. In fact, there was nothing abnormal in their behavior. They were just desperately reacting to her abnormal behavior.

She was an insomniac. So the first thing I did was to balance her meridians and instruct her to listen to a hypnosis tape, which I made especially for her, while having the Teragrams on her Chakras. This she did for seven nights. During those nights she slept and dreamed about herself and her problems. This way she was naturally helping herself to overcome many of her mental delusions. Next, I stimulated, toned and balanced her meridians, while focusing on her fear of rejection. This was followed up with counseling and full explanations about her state of mind. Two weeks later, she was to return for another session.

As I expected, she procrastinated. She could see herself beginning to change and she was terrified. She called me and informed me she wanted to stop coming. I explained to her what was happening, and convinced her to continue her treatment. She arrived looking in a state of extreme anger. She believed everyone was against her. She tried to make me agree with her. I placed her in hypnosis and let her know she could change without getting angry. That she could bargain with herself. She agreed to let anger leave her and replace it with the idea of bargaining with herself.

Next came another Crystal Acupuncture^sm treatment with the Teragrams. This time I stimulated her meridians to release anger. Her body twitched continually, as wave after wave of anger along with pain left her body. The Teragrams were constantly working, rebalancing the Chakras as I worked. The colors of her Aura were continually altering. It took two hours to get her into a stable state of relaxation. Once again, I placed her into hypnosis. This time, I made her a tape in which she was told to focus on her life in the future. She was told that now she was very positive and happy. In fact, the more she thought herself unhappy, the happier she became. Once again, she was awakened and sent home with instructions to listen to this hypnosis tape twenty-one times while the Teragrams are on her Chakras.

Two months later, she called me. "I can't stand living this life. I've got to end it. I need you to help me. I'm afraid I'll do something silly." Of course, I told her to come over right away.

That day she cried a lot. She cried her life away. Then I placed her in hypnosis and told her to relax. With circle therapy, I told her to think of the pain of her life and place it all in her right finger. When she did this, I told her to relax. Then I told her that each time she thinks of her pain, it will be less. We raised the finger several times, and each time the finger was not so high as the time before. Finally, I told her that no matter how hard she tried to think of the pain in her life, the happier she became. Now, I asked her to focus on her left hand. I asked her to think of a happy time and told her that her finger would rise on that hand. Her hand responded immediately. I then told her to relax. Then I told her to send any pain that was left in her right hand up through her brain, and down into her left hand where it would turn to joy. Her right finger immediately went up. At this point, I stimulated the meridians in the brain, as she refocused this energy to the left-hand finger. Once this finger rose, I had completed the connections between her left and right brain. My last command to her in hypnosis was that she should now see herself as completely healed. I then brought her out of hypnosis.

She was calm, and giggling. "What did you do to me?" she asked. I then explained to her how her left and right hemispheres of her brain had been in discord. She understood well. She felt better. Her emotional self was no longer suicidal.

One week later she returned for Teragram^{sm} Therapy. During this session, I lifted her vibration and refined her energies within the Five Bodies by using Crystal Acupuncture^{sm} to the last two toes, and then to the big toe. I used crystals that are in harmony with more spiritual vibrations. Tiger's Eye, Black Obsidian, Garnet, and Jade were most appropriate for this.

What followed for her was an immense and radical change in her outlook.

She became a different person. She found a new job, and eventually made a decision to break away from her negative family. As a result of her recovery, her family members came to me in their own time. I worked with each one, and they too are now happy. The last news I heard was that the family was back together again, and doing well.

A woman came to me with a cancerous lump in her breast. There was a history of cancer in the family and unfortunately, they had all died. My client was afraid she was going to follow her mother into an early grave.

I calmed her fears away by explaining how blocked energies can create tumors. I also gave her counseling about her attitude and the learned conditioned patterns of her life. She realized that the first thing she had to do was to stop thinking and acting on her negative emotions. She could see how she was just like her mother in many ways.

She had several Crystal Acupuncture^{sm} treatments, along with several Teragram Therapies while she was undergoing chemotherapy. During that time, she did not lose her hair, or feel sick like other patients. She was able to eat well, and still carry on a normal life. She would come directly from the hospital to me and then we would rebalance all her energies. The final result was a cure. She had many sessions with me, during which time I gave her advice, helping her to change her outlook on life. She is very active and happy now.

Unfortunately, I've had other clients who have not responded so well. Their need for attention was greater than their need for recovery. It is so easy to just settle for a hug and fool oneself into believing that all is well. These people were warned to change their emotions and their minds, but refused.

I watched the Crystal Acupuncture^{sm} treatments correct their energy flows, and then they would return one week later, all messed up again. Time and time again, I would unblock their energies, especially, those in the Etheric Body. Old mindsets were constantly reawakened and affirmed each time that they went home. They spent hours contemplating what was wrong with them and their lives. They lived in obsession. An obsession creates a depression, in which true feelings are repressed, and therefore, any desires to make changes become suppressed. These individuals were caught in a trap that they had created and could see no way out of it.

Several times in my life, I have had to use Crystal Acupuncture℠ to save someone's life. A friend of mine had a bad heart. She constantly told me that she would not live to be very old. One night she called me and told me that she was dying. She could see all her Spirit Guides and loved ones around her bed. I immediately rushed to her side. All her energies were practically on hold. I stimulated all the meridians and then followed up with tone and balancing.

As her energies began to harmonize once more, my own Spirit Guide, Chang, informed me that she needed more attention to her heart. He suggested that I use the Quartz crystal. With his help, I focused on her heart, while my husband placed his healing hands over her heart. She said she felt something happening inside her chest. I saw sparkles of gold in and around her Aura. After the healing was completed, we told her boyfriend to take her to the hospital.

That night she had surgery. The next day she was in intensive care, hooked up to many machines. I had come to give her another Crystal Acupuncture℠ treatment. I was just about to start when her doctor arrived. I explained what I was about to do. He informed me that he was very concerned for her. All the machines were showing him that she was not doing well at all. I then gave the treatment. He watched in amazement as each machine changed its rhythm taking her levels to the normal reading. When the treatment was finished, she awoke for the first time after her surgery. Her first words were. "Thank you Margaret, you saved my life." Her doctor then admitted that he had to agree.

During the operation, he had discovered that her carotid artery had a hole running through it. That hole was so perfect, it looked just as though something had drilled a perfect tunnel. Usually, arteries clog in different places, causing a winding pathway through the artery. When I explained how some crystals could bore a hole with energy that is heat turned into light, he began to understand the power of Crystal Acupuncture℠. More importantly, I knew that Master Chang had helped me do that to her. He had taken my energy and my husband's energy and condensed it into the flow that I was creating with Crystal Acupuncture^sm to make that hole. We must never forget the power of the Spirit World, and God.

Another friend was admitted to hospital for a simple operation. During the operation, his kidneys were destroyed by the anesthesia. He did not regain consciousness for several hours. As a result, they kept him in. Over the next few days he became disorientated and was unable to urinate. At that point, he was placed on dialysis. Then, they wanted to give him a kidney transplant. At this juncture in his ordeal, he called me.

I mixed him up a giant bottle of mixed herbal teas to reduce the swelling in the kidneys. When I arrived at the hospital, my friend's energies in the Five Bodies were at a very low ebb and flow. I immediately placed the Teragrams over his Chakras. His body told me that he had a fear of living life. This operation had brought that emotion to the surface along with a mental attitude to fight against all odds. His inner belief was that to live one had to struggle. With Aromatherapy oil, Reflexology and then Crystal Acupuncture^sm, I stimulated this negative energy and removed it from his Etheric Body. Then I harmonized the Five Bodies. I then stimulated the Spirit Body to increase the ebb and flow of the Five Bodies. This caused a general lift in his emotional outlook. He immediately began to talk about getting well.

At that moment, his doctor arrived. He wanted to put him on Cortisone. We both pleaded with him to wait for three days to pass. The doctor was clearly worried for my friend, and not at all impressed with my work. However, he had to comply with his patient.

My friend drank his tea, and in three days, he was able to urinate a little. I returned to give him another treatment along with more tea. By the end of the week, his kidneys were functioning enough for the doctor to release him from hospital. He continued to drink the tea for three months and to visit me one more time for another balancing. I am happy to report that he is now healthy and active and living his life to the fullest degree.

One lady had a speech problem. She was old and had acquired a reputation as a medium. Her speech was hindered by a self-imposed hypnotic suggestion that she could not speak. She had taken a regression session into a past life, were she had undergone a dreadful attack which had shocked her emotionally. Her mind then transferred this emotional fear into this life. When she came out of it, she could not speak. Therapy followed, during which time she struggled to speak again.

Finally, her quest took her onto a pathway of becoming a trance medium. In this state, she was relaxed and able to trust her Guides who spoke through her. Her words were clear and easily understood, unlike her voice when she was awake. I watched her as she channeled and saw how her energies flared and flowed as the Guides took over. Her Five Bodies harmonized and her voice improved. When her mind took over, the energies along her spine slowed, and dropped. She then struggled for her words. Her trance work was interesting and informative for those who listened. For me it was a clear lesson in watching how the mind controlled the energy flows of the body.

Later, I offered to work with her and try to help her speak again. We made an appointment and on that day, I took my friend and student with me. I felt that this was an exceptionally interesting case, and one that she could learn from by being involved.

I first used Reflexology to open up the Physical Body. During this time, she coughed and wheezed a lot, while constantly trying to explain herself. Remembering that all Chakras are divided into 5 equal parts for each of the Five Bodies, I let her talk, as the physical part of the Throat Chakra began to rotate. Then I used my crystals to stimulate the Etheric Body. I watched as the second part of the Throat Chakra began to rotate. Then I stimulated the Spirit Body and watched as the third part of the Chakra began to rotate. Her Higher Mind Body and Soul Body were already functioning well. The Chakra began to rotate at its healthy regular speed. She was still talking, and slowly her speech improved. I did not use hypnosis, as I knew her regression session had shown her to be super-sensitive to suggestions. Instead, I asked her to close down. She refused, informing me that she never closed down because her Spirit Guides always protect her. She was, nevertheless, amazed that she could speak much easier and more naturally.

Just then, her business partner came into the room. She spoke to him and he suddenly attacked me, telling me that I should not give her false hopes.

He stated that any help I may give her was really a selfish act to get her to trust me, so that I could take her church away from her.

I stood speechless. I had earlier offered to help her, because my Spirit Guides had told me that she was going to need help. I had no ulterior motives. She apologized for him, and then she rationalized how important he was to her. My friend and I watched all the work we had done dissipate as energy fell away from her. We knew that within a few hours she would, once again, be struggling to speak her words. We left, and one week later her partner died. I did offer to help her again, but she was too steeped in her own fear to let me help. As far as I know, she still struggles with her speech to this very day.

I have treated many individual cases of Bulimia, Anorexia, Agoraphobia, Claustrophobia, Vertigo, Schizophrenia, Paranoia, etc. The list goes on. All these types of illnesses are forms of obsession that have been created through fear of judgment. Often these people are full of judgment about themselves and the world, despite their own fear of being judged. In each case, it has always been necessary to deal with them in slow steps. It is rather like peeling off layers of an onion. Each layer is full of fear and anxiety, but little by little, the fear is released.

Each treatment with Crystal Acupuncture^{sm} is given first to release old mindsets along with negative emotions. Then hypnosis is used to give new suggestions. During that time, Crystal Acupuncture^{sm} and Teragram^{sm} Therapy must be used to harmonize and balance the ebb and flow of the energy in the Five Bodies. Each time the Five Bodies should be harmonized. It must be accepted that this harmony will shift as another layer of the onion is addressed.

In cases of extreme fear, I have seen my clients weekly, but as they improve, I make sure the sessions are more spread out. At first, it might be every two weeks, then once a month for six months and then once every two months etc. Eventually, my clients choose the times they want to come themselves. Every case is different and most interesting. It is important for a therapist to keep working within the natural pace of these clients. They will always present you with the problem. One needs to take one problem at a time and dissolve it. Eventually, there comes a time when they begin to trust the therapist and to develop a co-dependency. It is important to discourage this kind of bonding. This is an excellent time to begin spreading out the treatments, and a good time to begin serious counseling to redirect their thoughts and emotions into positive ideas about themselves and their lives.

When my children were young, they often brought me field mice, hedgehogs, birds, stray cats and dogs etc. Of course, the first thing I ever did was to heal them a little with my hands to calm them down. Animals do not understand anything you say, but they do feel everything you are. Household pets watch your actions and feel you. They learn through those associations what you are up to. In this way, they are no different from a toddler. They are also capable of seeing the pictures you create in your mind.

There was a time in England, when my Chihuahuas were itching with fleabites. I was watching the television and out of the corner of my eye, I saw them scratching themselves. I said to my husband, "I'd better do them." I got up and went to the kitchen to get the flea spray. My husband informed me that the dogs shot behind the sofa and were hiding. They obviously knew what I was going to do. They often saw me get up in the middle of watching television and on those occasions, they would simply watch me come and go or even follow me, especially when I went to find their food. This time, they clearly saw my mental pictures and had hidden.

When one is healing a wild animal, it uses its psychic senses to heighten its five physical senses. This is the way an animal lives. Humans tend to ignore this part of themselves, unless they decide to study metaphysics. When I'm healing an animal, I first use my psychic senses to connect and then send pictures of what I want to do. The animal is then allowed to sense my fear levels. It is important that I have none. It is the natural law of the animal world to surrender to the stronger. Now the animal is ready, if not willing, to let me approach. Sometimes it is necessary and sensible to make it impossible for the animal to hurt me. Cats have to be wrapped, in order to prevent clawing Some dogs have to be muzzled in order not to bite. These are sensible steps to take. However, they are not always necessary.

A healer can sense a way to communicate that they are no threat. Once that happens, healing can occur. However small the creature is, I first remove its fear and shock by sending my love and good thoughts into the animal. Then as it relaxes, I use Crystal Acupuncture^{sm} and stimulate the meridians. Later when the animal is more docile, I will return to balance the Five Bodies and the Chakras with Teragrams. Once the animal trusts me and its fear is erased, more sessions can be given. Healing is rapid, as the animal has no negativity.

Wild birds become tame in my hands, so I have to give them pictures of the wild and slowly prepare them to fly free. Tame animals do not require the freedom treatment. These animals often carry, pain, fear, anger and guilt. They have learned these things from humans. They need pictorial counseling and a lot of love. Slowly, they learn to make new picture associations and to trust again.

My own cat was one year old when she was given to me. She was already conditioned to be in fear and would not stay around any of the family members for long. She hated to be petted. One night, two young lads found her lying in the road. A vehicle had hit her. She was nearly lifeless with her tongue hanging out. Everyone in the family immediately gave her contact healing. She stirred a little and we knew she had enough energy in her to survive the journey to an overnight clinic for observation. No one knew if she had internal damage.

The next day found her very much alive, but physically she appeared to have a broken leg. We took her to the local Vet, who took an X-ray of her shoulder and leg. He had placed a dye in her leg, which showed clearly in the X-ray that her Femoral Nerve was severed. He advised amputation. I refused and he called me cruel. He informed me that she would never be able to use this leg and that it would have no feeling.

At home, I explored her body. Her spine and scapula were out of alignment, so I adjusted them, giving her body its natural line. Then I paid attention to her leg. I straightened the limb and strapped it to a spatula (tongue depressor). This made an excellent splint. Then, I sat with my Spirit Guides and focused on the end of the nerve. I manipulated the joint to bring the ends of the Femoral Nerve together and tied this part a little tighter. Then my Spirit Guides and I spiritually broke down the cells at the ends of the nerves, regrouped them together, and then reformed the nerve at the break. The family members spent the rest of the day taking turns to give hands-on healing.

The next day, I used Crystal Acupuncture[sm] to remove the shock of the accident, along with her fear of people. I then realigned her Five Bodies and with the use of one Teragram, rebuilt her Chakras. That was the easy part. Next came physiotherapy. I encouraged her to walk across the room with a splint on. As I held the weight of her body, I moved her leg forward to teach her how to walk on it again. Three days later, she could walk on this leg alone. A week had passed and it was time to remove the splint. She was lazy that day, spending most of her time licking the wound that was now exposed, where the nerve had been severed. Later that night, I used my crystals directly on the healing nerve to make sure that there was a neural connection with the brain.

Likewise I stimulated the brain and watched her neural reactions in the foot. All was well. Over the next five weeks, I used Reflexology and massage on her body, with Acupressure here and there to stimulate the nerve endings. Once a week she received a full Crystal Acupuncture[sm] treatment. By the end of six weeks, she was shaking her paw a lot and licking it. I knew then, that feeling was returning to the foot.

Now came the big day. I took her back to the vet. He informed me that his diagnosis had been correct and that she would never have feeling in that paw or be able to spread her claws. He took a needle and pricked her pad to prove his point. She clawed him. When he saw her reaction, he immediately rationalized that he had misdiagnosed. He even disbelieved his X-ray; saying there is no such thing as a miracle healing. Needless to say, I never went back to that vet again.

Earlier in my life, when I lived in England, a car also hit one of my Chihuahuas. He lay in a basket for two weeks without moving. Each day I applied my crystals to various parts of his body, and constantly had everyone in the family give contact healing. After these two weeks, we were beginning to think that this animal would have to be destroyed. Many friends were insisting this would be the kindest thing to do. My Spirit Guides had insisted otherwise, hence the Crystal Acupuncture[sm] treatments. On odd occasions I had found this animal's feces outside the basket and had wondered how it had got there because he could not walk.

Well, on the fifteenth day, he showed us all. He stood up on his front legs with his hips high above him, balanced and walked out of the basket onto the carpet, where he let himself down and went. This amazed us all. He certainly taught us that where there was a will there was a way. With renewed passion, I continued to heal this dog. Slowly over the next two weeks, the right hind leg began to hang a little lower. By then, we were use to seeing him walk around the house on two legs. Finally, he dared to put this third leg on the ground and walk on it. Everyone cheered. I continued to give healing treatments to all his meridians. Finally, in the sixth week, his last leg found the ground. His recovery was completed. He walked as well as any other dog and seemed to have no ill effects from the accident at all.

I owe a lot to that dog. By treating him, I was able to see, feel and know how each of the meridians is connected. Each stage of his recovery was a lesson for me, which I later went on to use with a man who had Multiple Sclerosis. Spirit told me that his brain was covered in pea-like shapes. I knew that My Spirit Guides had brought him to me to help me research further.

Over several sessions, I was able to improve his right side. He became strong and was able to stand on that leg again. His left side had not been worked. I was ready to start moving the energy on this side when he began to procrastinate about attending the sessions although they were free. Of course, I realized that he was afraid of his recovery. I also began to understand how important counseling and reprogramming was. At the time of healing this man, he was not receiving any counseling or emotional support. Small wonder, he stopped his treatment. He didn't know how to cope with the changes that were occurring.

My own journey in overcoming Parkinson's Disease was the most impressive way I learned about everything. Today, I am a living, walking example of successful healing. Every step of the way, my Spirit Guides showed me how to see what was happening to cause the disease. They showed me how to reprogram myself to change my attitude, my emotions, and to redirect my energies through new neural pathways that had not been used. As a result,

I have no shaking with very little loss of motor connections in the brain. I have discovered that I am dyslexic and sometimes word blind. This usually occurs when I am in my Beta state and tired. So long as I function in my Alpha state, that is my Psychic State I am able to communicate and write without problem. I am still investigating the power of the mind in relation to the energy flows of the brain.

I have also worked with Autistic children. These children are under eight years old and receptive to hypnosis. With the use of Crystal Acupuncture^{sm} and hypnosis tapes that are played nightly, these children have become conscious of their disabilities. They now keep their clothes on, use the potty, are learning to read and write and have longer attention spans. I also work with ADD and other compulsive disorders as well as treating those who are hearing and sight impaired. My insight into the energies of the mind is always astounding and truly enlightening. My Spirit Guides are always with me, helping me to understand my clients' problems and to effectively to help them the best way that I can.

Over the years, part of my research has been in dealing with addictive behavior and obsessive patterning. Whether these case have been dealing with alcoholism, illegal drugs, medications or mental illnesses that were originally brought on by erroneous behavior patterns created in adolescence. In every case where Crystal Acupuncture^{sm} was combined with other therapies including hypnosis, there has been tremendous growth in awareness on a spiritual level with, at worst, a significant change in habits. My clients/patients have 90% of the time greatly improved or completely cleared up. The few exceptions have been those who do not really wish to save themselves from their destructive habits.

CHAPTER 14

Spiritual Crystal Acupuncture^{sm}

A New Adventure

I have left Spiritual Crystal Acupuncture^{sm} until last. This is my latest adventure into the power of the crystals and the triangle shape. Many Metaphysicians have been playing with their ideas in trying to discover the value of the pyramid in healing. Research has shown that in a pyramid is a power point where energy is vibrating at such a fast rate that its vibration can sharpen a razor.

With this knowledge in mind, I set about discovering how an equilateral triangle has the same effect of healing as if you were able to be in the center of the pyramid. In meditation, I placed triangular shapes made of copper, silver and gold over my Third Eye Chakra and found that my meditations took on a different tone. They were more spiritual and more disconnected from the body. During my experiments in those days, I found I could astral travel easily.

I also tried drawing and then sitting in a triangle that I had marked out with wire in my back garden in England. Later I acquired my own copper pyramid. In all my experiments, I found that my energies were immediately altered. I quite naturally, drifted into a higher vibration, which allowed my Spirit Body to be more connected to my Physical Body, while in fact feeling more attached to the Spirit World and my Guides.

My interest in Spiritual geometry grew, and so my Spirit Guides explained to me how everything in the Universe is made of symmetrical shapes. These shapes attract one another. I played around with hexagonal, octagonal shapes etc., but the more I played, the more I found myself focusing on the triangle.

I began to work on myself with specially selected crystals, which had been cut into triangles for me. By placing one of these triangles upright on the Third Eye Chakra, it is possible to focus on your Spiritual reality, versus your Earthly reality. In Meditation, an awakening occurs that nearly always brings enlightenment. I was so impressed with this new therapy that I had triangles made especially for my students. These stones are also available for purchase from my company.

If in addition, a triangle is placed upright on each of the remaining four important Chakras, the Throat, Heart, Solar Plexus and Base, then an immediate lift in vibration is achieved. Anything can happen and does! You will naturally be drawn to the things that you need to know and to work on within yourself. As the triangles sit on the Chakras, each rotating core passes energy back and forth in and around the triangle, which creates a high intensity vibration that results in a shifting of the Five Bodies. Of course, you can focus on one Chakra at a time and select the triangle that you feel is most suitable for your meditation. You can also combine them with Teragram^{sm} Therapy. If you believe, you are in need of some great change that lies deep within you, it is a good idea to first place the triangle over the Chakra and then put the color Teragram of your choice on top. Relax and watch what happens. You may do several Chakras this way. I advise you not to try to do them all at once. It may be more than you can handle.

Remember that everything you see, hear, touch, taste and smell is affected by your history, where good and bad experiences have been recorded. If you choose to work with all five triangles and all five Teragrams at one time, you can be sure that those senses will be tested. You may hear Spirit voices, feel Spirits touching you, or find yourself back in past lives, remembering all the sensations of that life. If you are not prepared, this could scare the pants off you and do more harm than good. So, take it easy and walk slowly.

While there may be other stone triangles available, in my specially prepared Spiritual Crystal Acupuncture[sm] Kit, there are four pointed stones and five triangles. Each of these crystals has been carefully selected for their spiritual properties in being able to refine dense energy and redirect it according to desire. The following will give you some idea of which crystal is best to use:

SINGLE POINTS

TIGER'S EYE: (Black and yellow)

This crystal is capable of synthesizing the energies of Earth and the Sun. Our bodies are capable of absorbing these energies. Using this crystal will stimulate higher consciousness to awaken the Physical Body to its senses. It naturally clears away mental chaos, making room for the development of psychic ability and the opening of the Third Eye Chakra.

It naturally balances the energy flow of the Base (Root) Chakra, which in turn stimulates physical action. It also lifts the vibration of the Etheric Body, by harmonizing the Yin and Yang energy. It balances the Left and Right Brain, which generates awareness of a change in perception. It stimulates a desire to be fulfilled and to connect to The Oneness and Spirit Guides.

LEOPARD JASPER (Spotted brown and black)

This stone is the supreme nurturer. It provides protection by stimulating the light within, which in turn attracts the light beings of the Spirit World. It stimulates the Solar Plexus Chakra by aligning it with the other Chakras, which cause the Physical, Emotional and Mental Selves to balance. A state of inner harmony is
achieved. It stabilizes the Aura by cleansing and releasing negativity from the cellular-neuro-muscular memory. This allows rejuvenation of the Physical Body.

RHODONITE: (Pink with black marks)

This crystal is truly a blessing in itself. It balances the Yin and Yang energies and makes it possible to connect to the Universal Consciousness. It awakens spirituality and brings in a connection to receive unconditional love from God. This in turn stimulates the Heart Chakra to manifest one's greatest potential. It helps stimulate confidence and emotional contentment as well as developing intuitive abilities to receive guidance through connections with Spirit Guides.

SNOWFLAKE OBSIDIAN: (Black & white)

This crystal is one of the greatest presents that God has given us. It helps us to awaken to the unnecessary patterns in our lives, which hold us back in negativity. It quite naturally stimulates us to desire to make a change for the better. It helps in allowing a deep meditation state to occur and effectively lifts the vibration of the Five Bodies into a state of serenity. It can create a sense of isolation and observation of self, which then can directly lead to a focus on one's sensitivity around earthly love. It can then inspire the user to connect with the acceptance of self-love and self-beauty. A state of grace can then manifest.

THE TRIANGLES

PICTURE JASPER: (Brown with black lines)

This triangle will awaken memories in picture form from the past. It will stimulate old ideas to be recalled for review. In this state, one can release grief, negative thoughts, phobias and fears by facing their original cause. It also stimulates creative visualization to manifest the ability to tap into the unknown for insight and direction. This crystal stimulates appreciation of ones environment and motivates individuals to harmonize with others for a positive physical result. Business and family interactions become motivated towards success.

RED JASPER (Red)

This crystal is excellent for stimulating oneself to find obstacles that block one from seeing the truth about oneself. It increases perception and stimulates the desire to find a solution and a release of those blocks.

It also is an excellent tool for those who wish to remember their dreams. This stone stimulates the Third Eye, and the conscious mind to remember important aspects of those dreams and to recall them upon waking, or to returning into the dream and repeat it for further insight. It allows old memories to rise into the conscious mind for reevaluation and if necessary, elimination.

HEMATITE: (Silver-gray black)

This crystal calms the conscious mind and assists in awakening the *Spirit Mind* in meditation. It improves the right brain activity giving true focus and connection with Spirit Guides. It also utilizes the mind to balance the meridians of the Physical Body, and gives a calming effect on the nervous system. This crystal vibration gives true harmony to the Physical, Etheric and Spirit Bodies and creates a lifting of the three into a harmonic vibration, which allows unconditional love to flow. This stimulates inner peace and happiness, which in turn gives a strong sense of self-trust. Hematite also balances the magnetic forces of the physical form.

UNAKITE (Pink and Green)

This stone helps the Third Eye Chakra to open wide and focus on the ethereal planes of the Spirit World. It helps one to balance earthly emotions with spiritual ones, creating a need to rebirth. This rebirthing process moves earthly conditioning and physical blockages away. It then provides a doorway through which an individual can enter and awaken their inner awareness and to accept new experiences that ultimately result in a change of attitude and approach to life. Unakite allows connections to spirit entities in preparation for birth and rebirthing. A new mother can talk to her child-to-be, and a therapist can release a lost soul from the client's Aura, and direct them toward the Spirit World.

CALCITE: (Yellow)

This natural amplifier aids in helping the mind to remember spiritual experiences, such as astral traveling. It aids in allowing the conscious, sub-conscious, and deep-subconscious parts of the mind to connect with Spirit Guides and to recall all that occurred. It also helps the Spirit Body's physical experiences in the Spirit World to be remembered as a Physical

Body experience. This connection establishes a link for healing and a need to perfect ones way of life. Calcite polarizes and activates all the Chakras to cleanse and rebuild them without negativity. This is an excellent crystal for stimulating the Crown Chakra and connecting to God and Spirit Guides. It is a generator and stimulant that can effectively cause physical growth of new cells.

To begin using Spiritual Crystal Acupuncture[sm], you must first choose one or two of the pointed crystals and stimulate, tone and balance all your meridians by working the fingertip points. When you have done this, you will notice that you become relaxed and in a meditative mood. Select the triangle that you have decided to work with and place it on the Chakra that you have chosen to focus on. If you wish to add a Teragram, do so. Now relax and meditate.

As you experiment with each crystal point and use a different triangle, you will have a different experience in your meditations. As there are many combinations of ways to use the crystals and your Teragrams, you will find you have many years of wonderful meditative states ahead of you. Remember that each Chakra needs to be worked on separately at first. When you become more familiar with your crystals and the effects they have on you, you will be able to handle more crystals at one time. Ultimately, you may be able to handle both the triangles and the Teragrams on all your Chakras as you lay and meditate.

If you wish to work on the Crown Chakra with a triangle, then it will be necessary to sit upright, or find a way to stick it to your hair. I have used a piece of sticky tape, which has not affected the potency of the crystal. If you do decide to sit up, then make sure your back is well supported. Once you move into a deep state of meditation, you will no longer be aware of your body, but if the body is uncomfortable in the beginning, it will prevent your reaching this great state of meditation.

The Spleen Chakra is always in need of rebalancing. It is quite in order to use your crystal points on this Chakra, and rotate the crystal until you feel this Chakra vibrating. If you wish to hold a triangle over this Chakra, then do so. It will of course, lift your vibration.

If you are a therapist, you may have occasion to use Spiritual Crystal

Acupuncture^sm on a client who is paranoiac, in hysteria, or panic. You can even use this therapy on a client who is unconscious. Simply place the triangles over the Main Chakras and then put the crystal point into the center of the triangle and rotate clockwise. These two crystals have a combined energy force that will calm a person down, and awaken them to reality. It will consciously help them to deal with their situation and to realize where they are. In coma cases is necessary to place the triangles point down, in order to draw the spirit back into the body and into waking consciousness. This method usually results in the client waking up around three days later. Then Crystal Acupuncture^sm with Teragram^sm Therapy should be given, with a final five minute treatment with the five triangles pointing upward on the central core of each Chakra to stimulate new growth and new ideas for living life.

It is also possible to integrate your regular Crystal Acupuncture^sm points with the triangles. Feel free to explore with them and discover their power. Even wear them on a chain. The more you experiment, the greater your understanding will be.

Many of my students are now writing to me. Their reports are exhilarating. They tell stories of successes where medical care has failed. They all speak of how powerful my therapies are. I hope you will write to me and let me know how you are doing with both your Crystal Acupuncture^sm and Spiritual Crystal Acupuncture^sm Therapies combined. I am also interested in hearing stories about how Teragram^sm Therapy has changed people's lives.

CHAPTER 15

Working With Clients

A fter having read this book, I am sure you may find yourself thinking "there is so much to do and I'm not sure where to start!" This Chapter is dedicated to helping you to get that start. First, of course, you must acquire your stones. It is quite in order to have a collection of your own crystals; however, you may find it difficult to find all the crystals that are used in my kits. If this is the case, you may obtain them from my company.

Having read this far, you now understand how important it is to have a place of work that is quiet and nurturing. Make sure that you are in a good mood and that you clearly understand the problems that your client/patient is presenting to you. Once you are ready to begin work, remember to focus in prayer or meditation to your Guardian Angels/Spirit Guides and to tell your client/patient to do likewise. Once this is done, both you and your client/patient should visualize all your days' negativity leaving the body through the feet.

A simple visualization of being in the shower, and watching all your dirt running down your body into the drain is sufficient. However, if you have your own method, please feel free to use it. At this point, it is also a good thing to remember God and be receptive to receiving His love. Play an appropriate musical meditation tape quietly.

No matter what is wrong with your client/patient, it is always appropriate to talk your client into a relaxation mode. Simply guide them to focus on the body and to relax the muscles.

Here is a simple relaxation technique:

> **Feel/sense/think (word used depends on the type of person you are helping) the top of your head and sense all the hairs that are growing on your scalp. Take a deep breath and let your brain relax. Now sense your face, and allow all the muscles around your eyes, nose, ears and mouth to relax. Take a deep breath. Relax. Attune to your neck. Let all the muscles, both inside and outside, relax, especially the back of the neck and shoulders. Relax. Focus now on your chest. Watch yourself breathing and let your back relax all the way down to your tailbone. Relax. Take another deep breath and feel your abdomen relaxing. Let your hips and thighs relax now and feel your knees and lower legs relaxing at the same time. Now feel how your feet, especially the toes are relaxing as you let all the muscles throughout your body relax. Take a deep breath. Relax.**

If you are ready to place the Teragrams on the Chakras, you may like to guide your client/patient to feel you placing them in position. As you do this, ask them to open the Chakras by visualizing a small circle of light, opening up and expanding to become a ring of light. Another method is to ask them to relax their muscles in the areas of the Chakras, while saying to him/her, "I open this Chakra". You may have your own method. Whichever way you choose to work with them, remember that once the Chakras are open, your client/patient is going to be very receptive to you and the healing that you are giving. They will be very vulnerable and extremely receptive to everything you say and do.

During the time that you are helping your client/patient to relax and open the Chakras, you could choose to do Reflexology to the feet or hands. Reflexology stimulates the meridians to open by causing a series of impulses, which will unblock surface trauma, resulting in temporary relief. This will automatically take your client/patient into a more relaxed state.

Watch your client/patient for rapid eye movement and a general change in their breathing pattern. This is a perfect time to remind them of their desire to heal themselves. They are, of course, in hypnosis and open to suggestions that will help them heal. Remind them that you are about to use Crystal Acupuncture[sm] and ask them to watch or sense themselves feeling energy flowing. Do not worry if they do not respond or tell you they cannot feel. They will be watching everything you do on some level or other.

Now, using the Quartz crystal, hold it at the center of the tip of the toe, approximately 2mm. away from the nail, while holding the toe with fingers from your other hand. Allow your energy to flow from your hand into the crystal. Be receptive to the energy flows of your client/patient. If they are receiving your energy, you will feel heat and energy leaving your hands. If the client/patient is not receptive, then impound this Acu point.

Remember that impounding an Acu point will force energy along the meridian, causing any blocks to disperse. If there is a block on the meridian, the hand that is holding the crystal will feel energy building as static electricity manifests in the wrist and arm, causing a tingling sensation. After five or six impounds, note how the tingling sensation ceases as the client's/patient's energy begins to flow. Once the energy is flowing, hold the crystal on the point again and wait for a return of flow into your other hand. Both hands will tingle when the energy flow is complete.

Now, hold the crystal still on the Acu point to tone and balance this meridian. Then rotate the crystal on the point and watch your client for obvious neuro-muscular responses, such as coughing, itching, twitches etc, while at the same time, noting any ideo-motor responses that may be surfacing from the subconscious. These movements are usually very slight, but obvious, such as an eyebrow raise, or a little toe spread. Remember that everything you see is in some way a part of their cellular-neuro-muscular memory, which is releasing old history tapes.

If you are a Psychic, you may be experiencing empathetic symptoms and memories of your own. Try to isolate the message you are receiving from their body, and note it for further discussion later. Such an example might be a sense of tension around the head and a deep-seated feeling of fear of the unknown. This will give insight into the client's state of mind and their attitude towards life.

Continue to perform Crystal Acupuncture^sm on the top of each toe on this foot. When you have finished this foot, treat the other foot in the same manner. There is no rule as to which foot should be treated first. I tend to treat the left foot first to stimulate the feminine side of the higher self, and the clarity of thought in the brain. Once I have this part of the body flowing, it becomes easier to move more energy in the Physical Body. However, everyone is different, and you must rely on your intuition, which of course, is your spiritual psychic self, to select the correct foot. Do not doubt your choice. Trust that it will always be the correct one. Do likewise with the hands and any other part of the body that you feel needs treatment.

Now that you have stimulated, toned, balanced and released energy in each meridian of the Physical Body, it is time to release old memories, emotions and thoughts from the Etheric Body. Select the stone of your intuitive choice and treat each toe/finger in the same manner as before. Be prepared for anything during this time.

Your client/patient may cry, shout, yell, scream, or simply tighten their jaw and resist releasing. While all this is occurring, they may fidget, fumble, scratch, twitch etc. etc. All this is part of the ideo-motor responses of release. At times, when appropriate, ask your client/patient to take deep breaths and think of releasing negative energy through the foot Chakras into the ground.

Try to note any pictorial images that arise as you heal. These are silent ways you interpret the state of your client/patient. If you find yourself thinking or feeling a need to say a *key* word such as *Mother*, then ask them to say this word to themselves over and over again, or repeat it aloud several times. This will stimulate associations, which the subconscious will bring to the surface of the body. Instruct the client/patient to continue deep breathing, while watching the images appearing and disappearing. Do not allow them to attach any importance to these images. Remind them that this is simply old history being released. With each release, rotate the crystal on the Acu point to balance and realign the meridian.

My students have often asked me "How will I know when to stop doing this part of the treatment." The answer is quite simply, that both the client/ patient and the healer always come to a moment of union, when both feel, "Enough is enough." That, of course, is the time to cease stimulating the point. Each point may be stimulated four or five times. After that, it becomes overload. I often find only two or three times quite sufficient. Once each foot has been worked on, it is time to harmonize the Chakras. The client/patient's mind is always involved in everything that is occurring, even if they are asleep.

I often use Aventurine or Sodalite to calm and redirect energies as they pass through the mind. Even my own thoughts are transmitted in the form of energy into a subconscious and deep-subconscious mind. If I think and feel love for my client, the client through Psychometry will feel this. They will feel this love and allow it to flow through their body. If I think, "You are safe," they will receive the feeling of safety. Because they are in a hypnotic state, any words, feelings or thoughts given to them will help their energies to flow productively into a state of grace and harmony. At this point healing begins to occur.

If the Teragrams are not already on the body, they should now be set in position. The healer should ask the client/patient to focus on the Chakra being treated and to visualize it rotating. I often ask my clients to visualize the hands of a clock moving around to the right, and then as they watch, noticing how the hands move faster and faster until they can no longer see the hands spinning round. When this occurs, the Chakra is usually spinning correctly. Another way to help them visualize, is to think of a child's spinning top that is wobbling around. Ask them to work the top so that it spins faster and faster until you can hardly see it rotating.

Each Chakra should be rebuilt in this way, and then harmonized with one another. To do this, the healer must put one hand on one Chakra and another hand on another Chakra. The Teragrams remain in place. Because the healer's Hand Chakras are wide open, energy flows from the healer, through the Teragram and on down into the Chakra. There it is spun around and then passed on in the energy flow of each body to the next Chakra. As each Chakra balances, the healer will feel equal heat and tingling sensations in both hands, which is a sure sign that both Chakras are fully functioning and in harmony with one another.

The healer should start with the Base (Root) Chakra and harmonize it with the Solar Plexus Chakra. Then the Solar Plexus Chakra should be harmonized with the Heart Chakra, then the Heart Chakra with the Throat Chakra. The Throat Chakra should then be harmonized with The Third Eye Chakra. Finally, the Crown Chakra should be harmonized with all the other Chakras. This can be done by placing one hand on a Teragram which is held at the center of The Crown Chakra, while the other hand holds a Teragram either over the pubic bone, or more ideally, between the inner thighs. If the client is agreeable, the Teragram should be held about two inches below the private parts. It will still effectively balance the flow of energy between the two hands of the healer. If the healer aligns the Chakras in this way, it will ensure a good flow of energy up and down the neural spine. This in turn will send energy though every one of the Five Bodies and to every part of the Physical Body.

Lastly, the Spleen Chakra should be harmonized to the other six Major Chakras. Once again, the healer should select two Teragrams. One Teragram should be held over the right front part of the Chakra, while the other Teragram should be held over the left rear part of the Chakra. As the healer sends energy from the front to the back, so the hand at the rear will send energy back along that Chakra to the front. When it becomes balanced, harmonized and polarized, both hands of the healer will tingle with static electricity. The Teragrams may be held in the palms of the hands up against the spleen Chakra at both ends. The palms should then rotate the Teragrams to activate the DNA memory to restore power in the Solar Plexus Chakra where heat can soon be felt.

If the healer has sense of a need to even out layers of the Aura, then the Teragrams can be methodically moved around the human form without touching. It may be necessary to be as much as two to three feet away from the Physical Body. Once the Aura is built up, Psychometry will help the healer to feel a resistance in the Aura when a hand tries to pass through it about three feet away from the physical form.

Now, all that is left to do is to ask the client/patient to close the Chakras beginning with the Base (Root) Chakra. Ask them to visualize a large white ring of light over each Chakra while pulling in and tensing the muscles in that area. Tell them to watch the ring getting smaller and smaller until they only see or sense a speck of light. Once this is done they can relax and move on to the next Chakra. When the Base, Solar Plexus, Heart, Throat, Third Eye Chakras are closed, help them to become aware of their Crown Chakra. This Chakra should never be completely closed. Ask them to visualize it closing, rather like a lady's fan closing until it is only three inches open. Now ask them to visualize it spinning clockwise on their head, forming a funnel that connects them to God and their Spirit Guides.

The Spleen Chakra should then be balanced. Ask the client/patient to sense this Chakra and to visualize or sense that they are looking at a set of scales with numbers one through one hundred. Ask them to find the indicator and bring it to fifty. Once this is achieved, the Chakra is balanced. Now ask them to stretch their sides upwards and to think "Close".

Finally, the Hand and Foot Chakras need to be closed. Simply ask them to make a fist and then wriggle the toes, while saying "Close" to him/herself. This is an automatic direct command that the conscious mind understands and will comply.

The above treatment is the beginning of creating great changes in a person. A follow up counseling session is necessary. If a person has a specific physical complaint, then a more focused treatment will be necessary. The toes and hands can still be worked on as suggested above, but emphasis must also be made on the meridian the flows through the part of the body that is ailing. If necessary, the Acu point directly over the afflicted area should be stimulated, toned and balanced as well as released. In *The Book of Crystal Acupuncture*^{sm} *and Teragram*^{sm} *Therapy Diagrams*, I have illustrated diagrams that show the points, which should be worked for various maladies.

The above treatment is a basic treatment that will help everyone. Spiritual Crystal Acupuncture^{sm} can also be used during this treatment. Simply place the triangles of your choice over the Chakras while working the points. Remember that you can place a Teragram on top of the Triangles for maximum effect. Be sure, however, that your client/patient is ready for a radical change. Often, a client wants to be healed but is psychologically unprepared for the changes.

Your crystals are your friends. They all have characters of their own. When you work with them and become familiar with the techniques, you will feel as though they are a part of you. When you drive your car, you do not think about every move you make. You just do what is necessary to get yourself about. Using your crystals will be just the same. You will grow to know instinctively which crystals you want to use and exactly where and how you want to use them.

When you set up your practice, remember that cleanliness is next to Godliness. Make sure that the room in which you practice has clean accessories and that your crystals and Teragrams are washed between treatments on each client. Make sure you use warm soapy water that has an anti-bacteria formula. You should always provide cotton or disposable gowns for your clients as well as fresh linen and towels. Piped music with a comfortable décor will help them to relax. Enjoy being a therapist and your clients will enjoy you.

My research over the years has never ceased to amaze me. Time and time again, I have thanked my Spirit Guides for making me aware of these three wonderful therapies. The emotional joy of my work is priceless, as I see client after client recover or greatly improve their condition. I am now currently sharing my knowledge with my students who are by their questions pushing me deeper into my research. I constantly remind myself how nebulous, and yet so obvious, are the brain waves, which control us, causing our bodies to be ailing. While I have found and taught about many patterns within our ways of thinking and feeling that result in negative control, I am still in search of a way to promote positive conditioning in a practical earthly sense, that will allow a new generation to manifest without fear of survival.

At this time of printing I am currently researching my new therapies ***TrinityStone^{sm} Healing and "Core" Teragram^{sm} Therapy.*** Trinity Stone Healing^{sm} releases audio negative programming from the cellular-neuro-muscular memory that has been encoded throughout life and prior to birth. These specially chosen large triangles when placed on the central core of each Chakra, will while listening to music, dialogue etc, release bad programming and heighten good tonality in positive focus, stimulating acceptance of self and the world. It is my intention to write a book about this therapy soon.

"Core" Teragram^{sm} Therapy releases conscious and unconscious memories with the use of three new Teragrams in colors black, teal and burgundy. The black Teragram can only be placed on the Base (Root) Chakra or Solar Plexus. The other two integrate between the Solar Plexus, Heart and Throat Chakras. With a special CD I have made a client/student can change their point of view about many issues that emotionally been blocked.

As the years pass, I have never ceased to be amazed by the new information and practices that my Spirit Guides give me and I am grateful for every opportunity to share this information with others. I hope that by reading this book you will find a way to enjoy using crystals to make your life whole and perfect.

If you are interested in becoming a certified Crystal Acupuncturist and Teragram Therapist, please feel free to contact me. I am always teaching somewhere in the world and will be happy to include you in my workshops. If you simply want to heal yourself, then I can be there for you too. I also earnestly suggest that you, send for ***The Book of Crystal Acupuncture*^{sm} *and Teragram*^{sm} *Therapy Diagrams, The Way to Oneness, The Rejection Syndrome,*** and ***Pro-Life, Pro-Choice, Pro-Spirit.*** Each of these books is filled with a great deal of information, which will help you understand yourself in a better light and therefore help you to be a greater healer.

You can write to Margaret Rogers Van Coops, Ph.D. DCH(IM): c/o Sumaris Enterprises, 321 Farallon Dr., Lake Havasu City, AZ 86403, USA. or Email: drmargaretrvc@gmail.com. If you want to know more about our products and services, our website is www.sumariscenter.com

I know that whatever you do, you will find your life improving as you use these therapies. Remember, always "Walk in the Oneness."

APPENDIX

The Laws Of Karma
Stages Of Loss
Soul Fears
The Aura
The Physical Body Energy Flow
The Etheric Body Energy Flow
The Spirit Body Energy Flow
Higher Mind Body Energy Flow
The Soul Body Energy Flow
Major And Minor Chakras Treatments
Major And Minor Chakras Frontal And Lateral
Chakra Rotation And Cone Structure
L-R Brain
Body Zones
Treatment For Your Pet

THE LAWS OF KARMA

1. No fragment may impose its will on another at anytime on any level

2. Each fragment shall be responsible for all it creates in positive and negative actions

3. Each fragment shall share itself with all other fragments in unconditional love

4. Each fragment shall attract like in the mirror image, either in opposition or support for growth without judgement

5. Each fragment shall, in unconditional love, surrender to The Creator

STAGES OF LOSS

1. Anger arises and blame and shame are bandied about in rejection and sorrowful tears

2. Tears flow as abandonment and misery compound sorrow and despair in obsessive failure

3. Failure generates a need for success and comfort, which gives birth to desire and bargaining

4. Bargaining opens a door to new awarenesses and new beginnings that herald the presence of joy and love

SOUL FEARS

*A fragments journey in
embodiment must face and use
these fears and overcome them*

Fear of Ascension - Fear of Success

Fear of Descending - Fear of Failure

*Fear of Separation - Fear of being
cast out*

*Fear of Assimilation - Fear of being
lost*

Fear of Love - Fear of becoming God

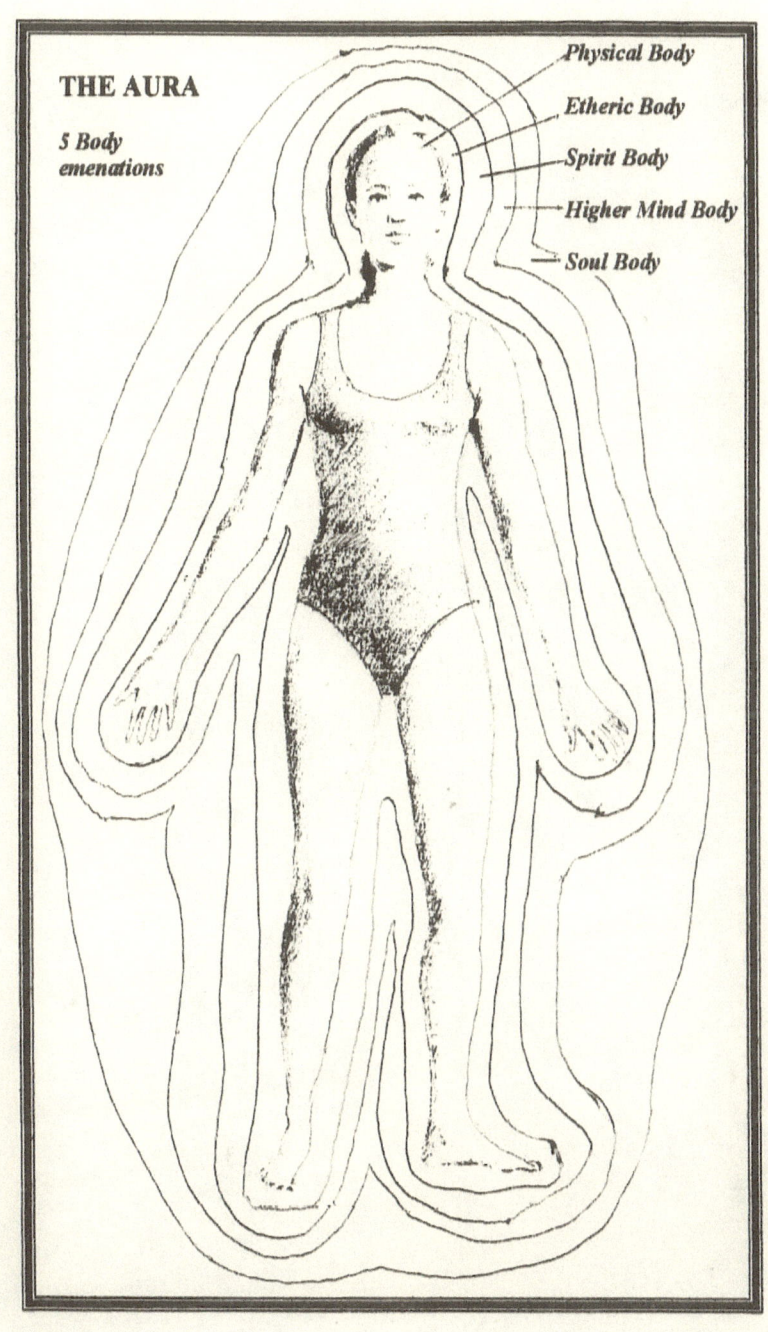

THE AURA

5 Body
emenations

Physical Body
Etheric Body
Spirit Body
Higher Mind Body
Soul Body

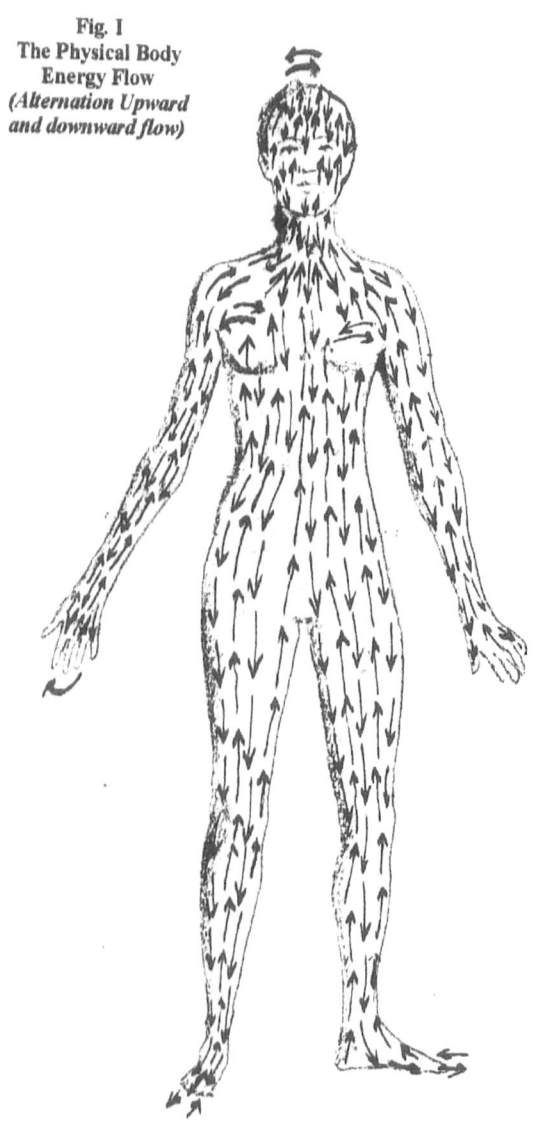

Fig. I
The Physical Body
Energy Flow
*(Alternation Upward
and downward flow)*

150

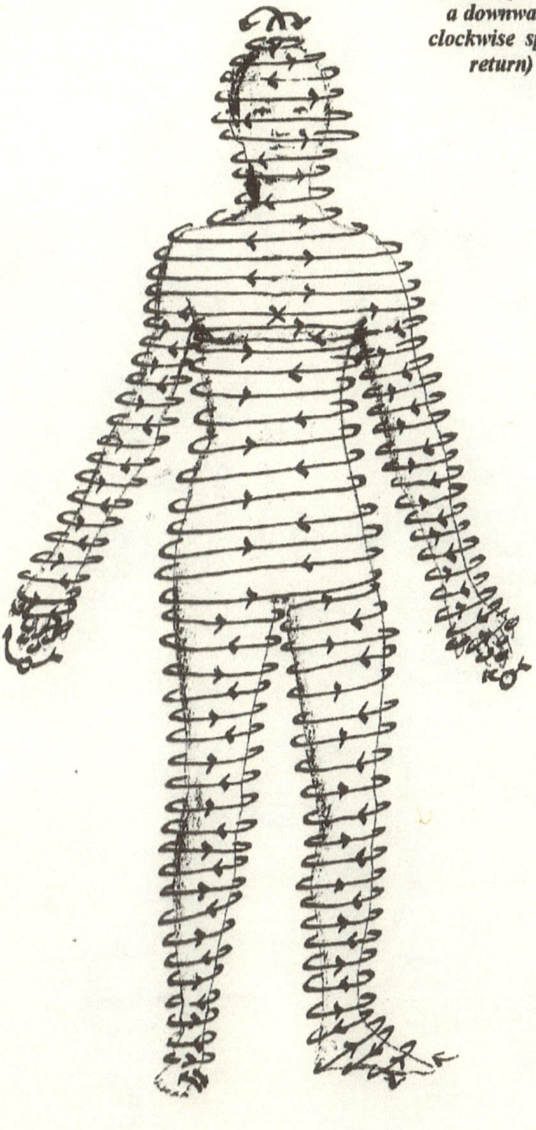

Fig. II
The Etheric Body
Energy Flow
(Ascending anti-clockwise spiral with a downward clockwise spiral return)

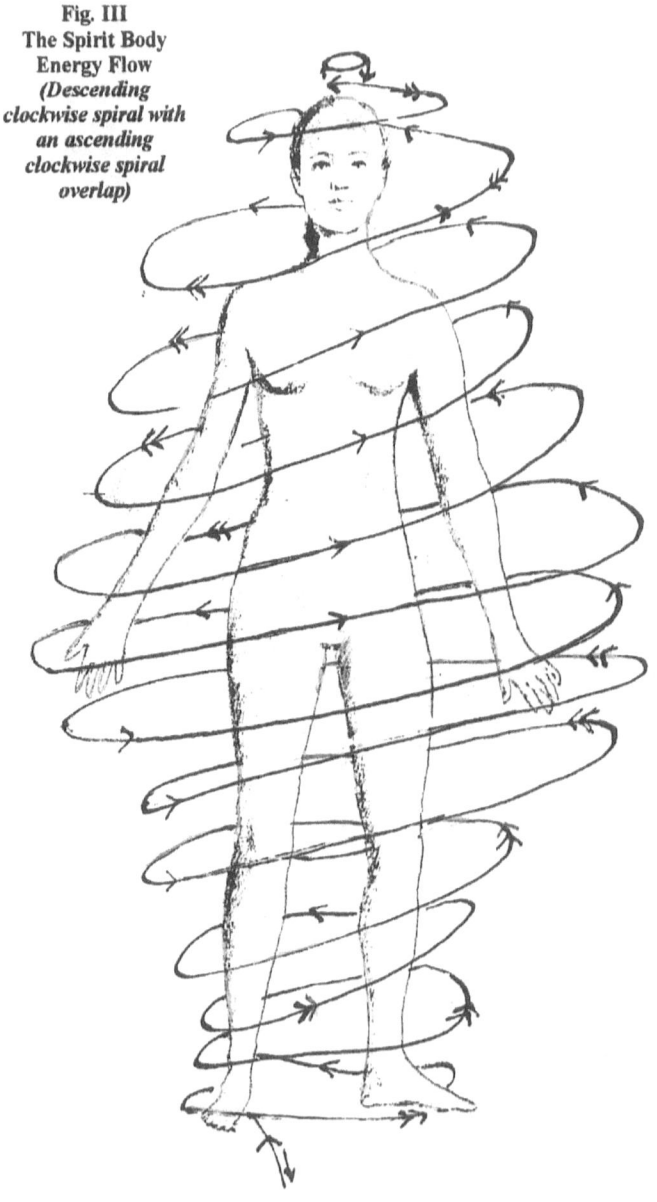

Fig. III
The Spirit Body
Energy Flow
*(Descending
clockwise spiral with
an ascending
clockwise spiral
overlap)*

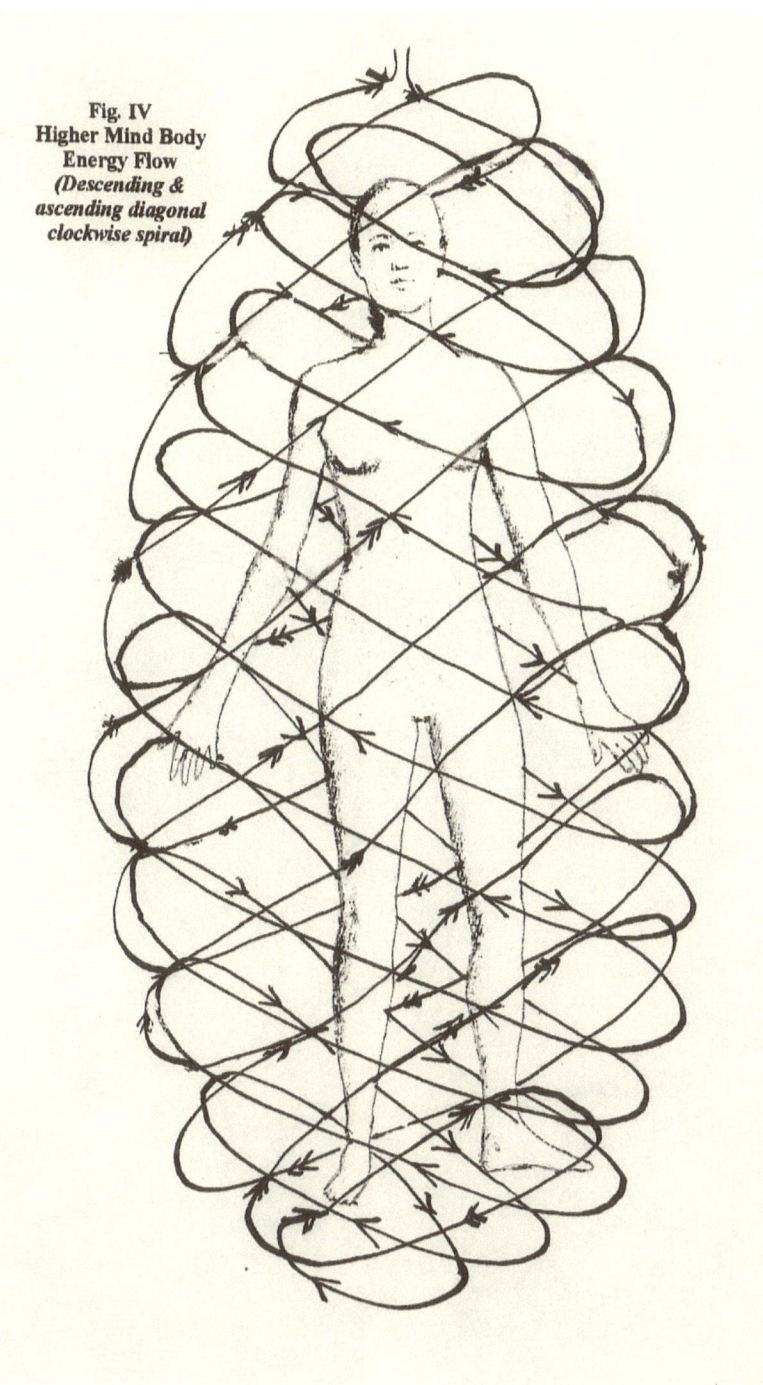

Fig. IV
Higher Mind Body
Energy Flow
*(Descending &
ascending diagonal
clockwise spiral)*

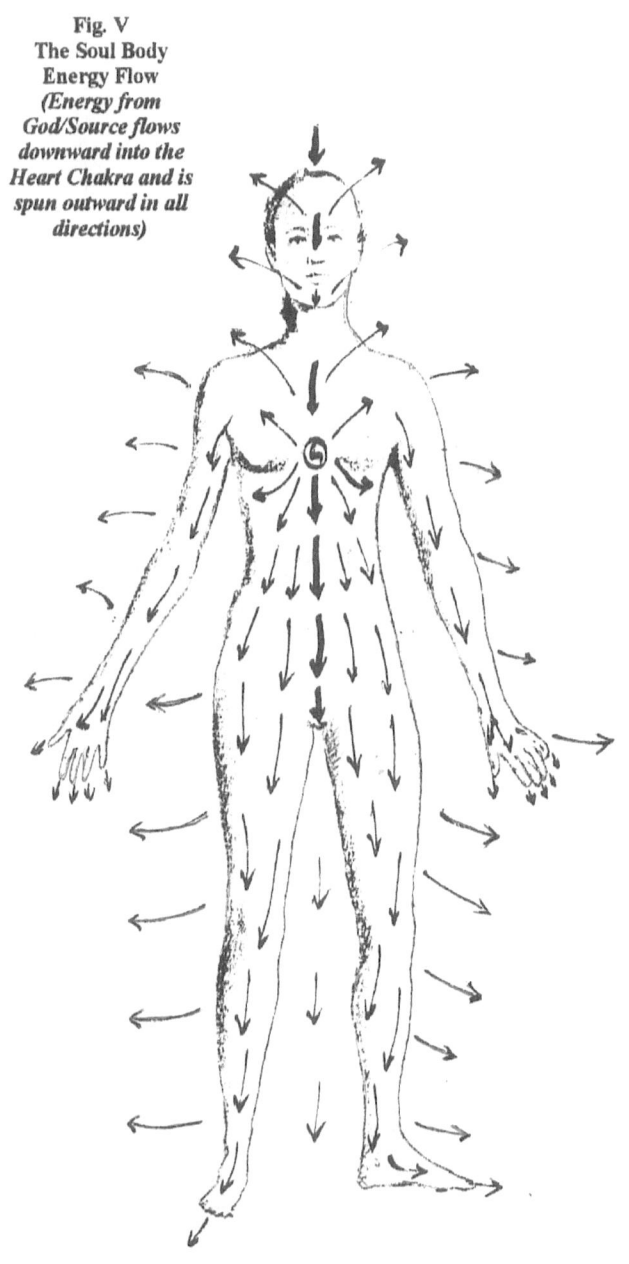

Fig. V
The Soul Body
Energy Flow
(Energy from
God/Source flows
downward into the
Heart Chakra and is
spun outward in all
directions)

MAJOR & MINOR
CHAKRAS

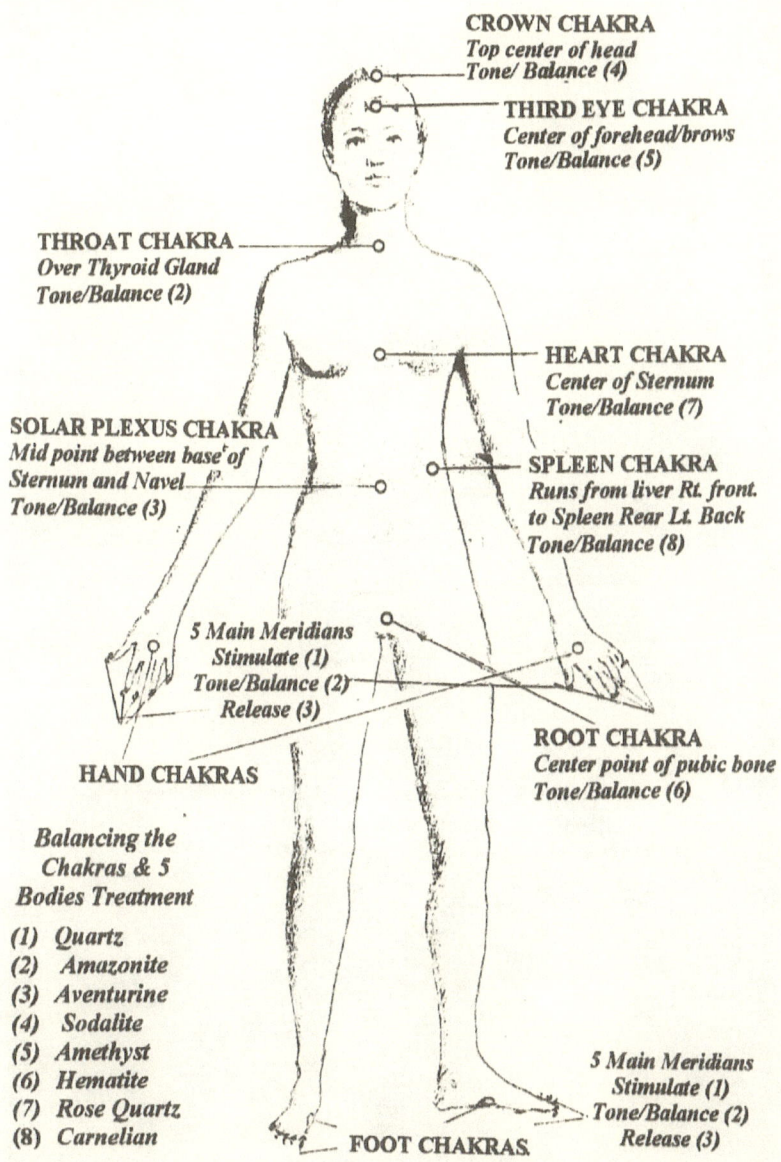

CROWN CHAKRA
Top center of head
Tone/ Balance (4)

THIRD EYE CHAKRA
Center of forehead/brows
Tone/Balance (5)

THROAT CHAKRA
Over Thyroid Gland
Tone/Balance (2)

HEART CHAKRA
Center of Sternum
Tone/Balance (7)

SOLAR PLEXUS CHAKRA
Mid point between base of
Sternum and Navel
Tone/Balance (3)

SPLEEN CHAKRA
Runs from liver Rt. front.
to Spleen Rear Lt. Back
Tone/Balance (8)

5 Main Meridians
Stimulate (1)
Tone/Balance (2)
Release (3)

HAND CHAKRAS

ROOT CHAKRA
Center point of pubic bone
Tone/Balance (6)

Balancing the
Chakras & 5
Bodies Treatment

(1) Quartz
(2) Amazonite
(3) Aventurine
(4) Sodalite
(5) Amethyst
(6) Hematite
(7) Rose Quartz
(8) Carnelian

5 Main Meridians
Stimulate (1)
Tone/Balance (2)
Release (3)

FOOT CHAKRAS

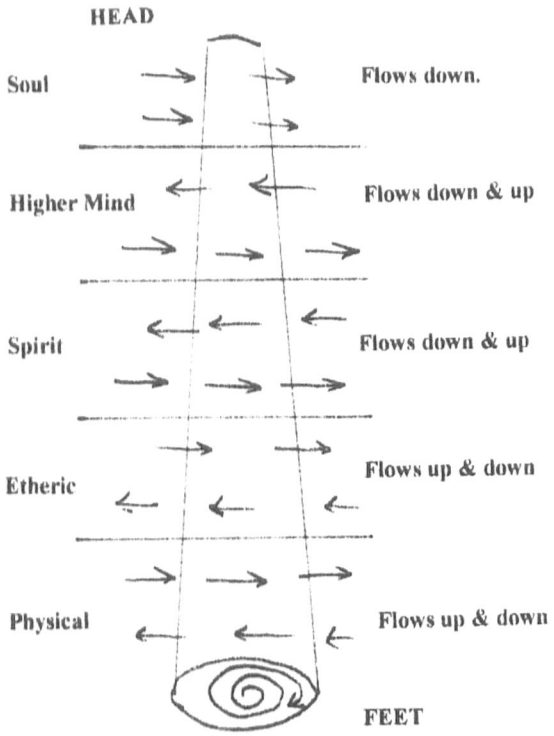

HEAD

Soul — Flows down.

Higher Mind — Flows down & up

Spirit — Flows down & up

Etheric — Flows up & down

Physical — Flows up & down

FEET

Rotation Of The Base Chakra

N.B. Third Eye, Throat, Heart, Solar Plexus Chakras
flow from front to back & back to front.
Crown Chakra flows from head to Base Chakra & up

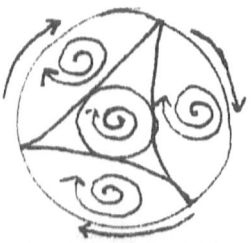

Four Cones Within
The Base Chakra

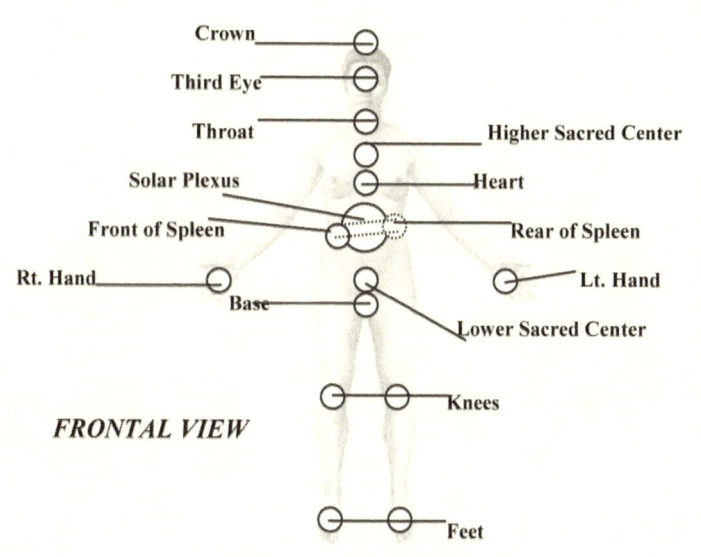

Crown

Third Eye

Throat

Higher Sacred Center

Solar Plexus

Heart

Front of Spleen

Rear of Spleen

Rt. Hand

Lt. Hand

Base

Lower Sacred Center

Knees

FRONTAL VIEW

Feet

MAJOR & MINOR CHAKRAS

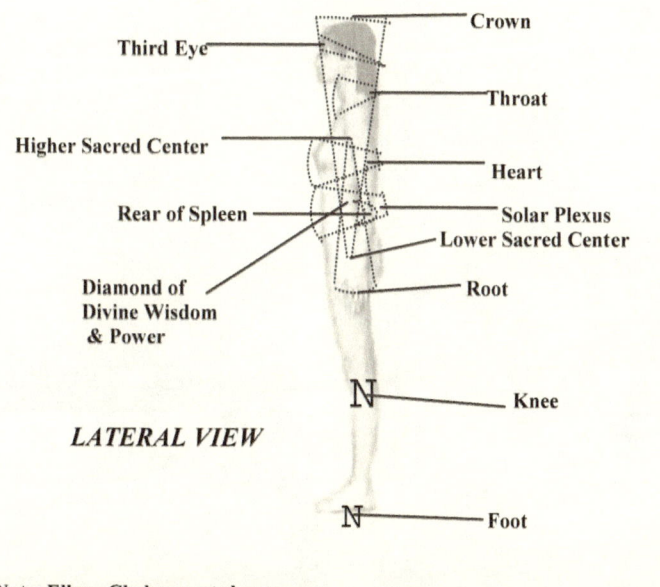

Crown

Third Eye

Throat

Higher Sacred Center

Heart

Rear of Spleen

Solar Plexus

Lower Sacred Center

Diamond of
Divine Wisdom
& Power

Root

Knee

LATERAL VIEW

Foot

Note: Elbow Chakras not shown

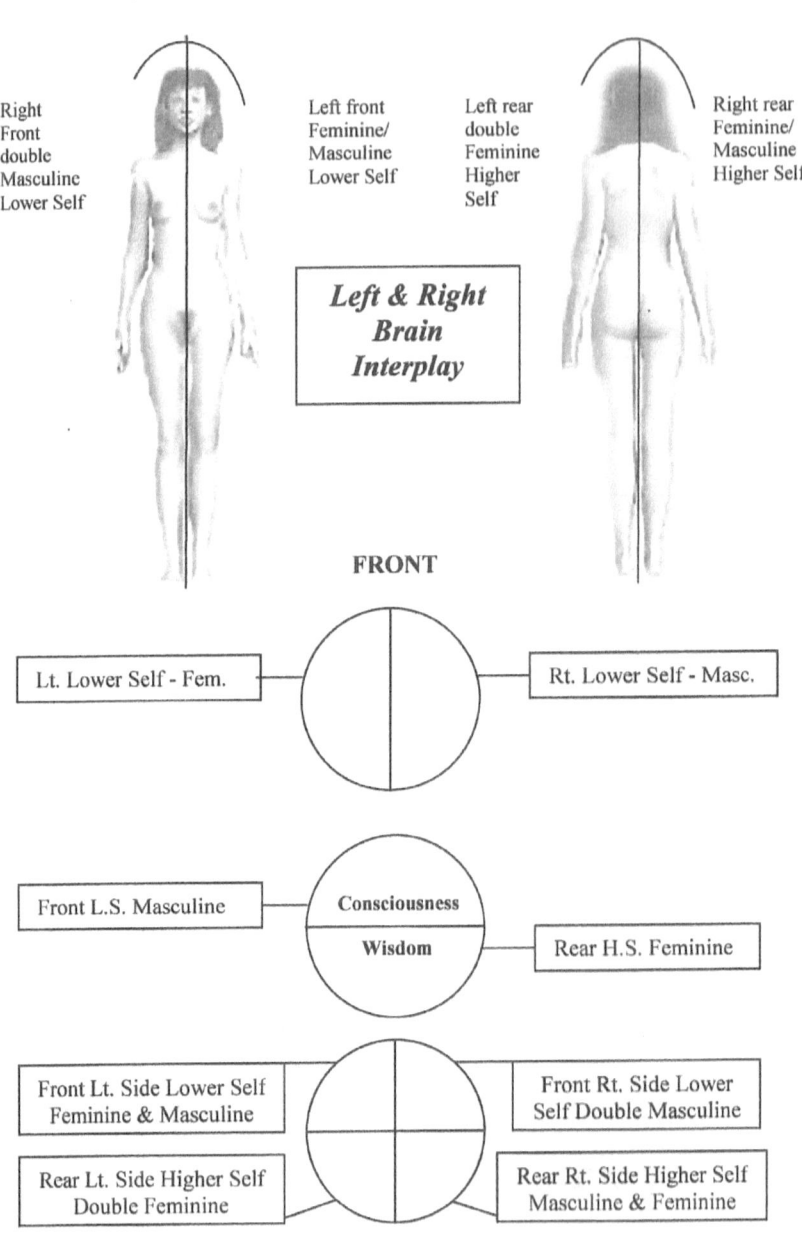

Right
Front
double
Masculine
Lower Self

Left front
Feminine/
Masculine
Lower Self

Left rear
double
Feminine
Higher
Self

Right rear
Feminine/
Masculine
Higher Self

**Left & Right
Brain
Interplay**

FRONT

Lt. Lower Self - Fem.

Rt. Lower Self - Masc.

Front L.S. Masculine

Consciousness

Wisdom

Rear H.S. Feminine

Front Lt. Side Lower Self
Feminine & Masculine

Front Rt. Side Lower
Self Double Masculine

Rear Lt. Side Higher Self
Double Feminine

Rear Rt. Side Higher Self
Masculine & Feminine

REAR

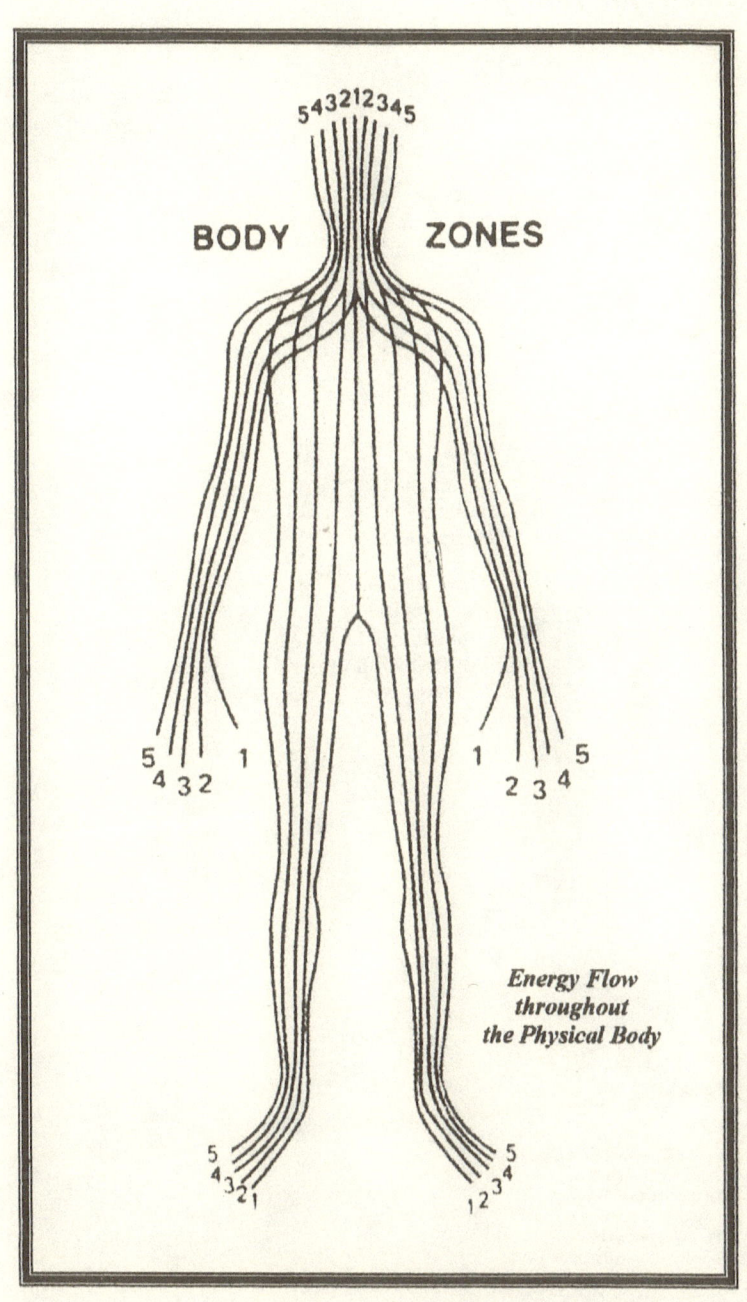

BODY ZONES

543212345

5 4 3 2 1   1 2 3 4 5

Energy Flow
throughout
the Physical Body

5 4 3 2 1   1 2 3 4 5

Treatment for your pet

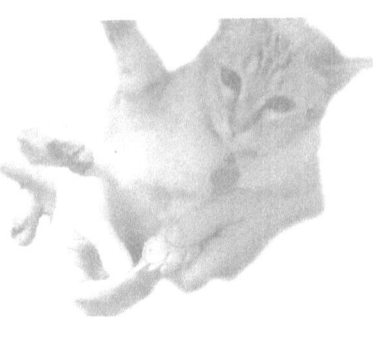

Amethyst (for general healing)
A crystal should be placed
on each pad 1 mm. behind the
claw. First impound, then rotate
& hold to achieve balance.

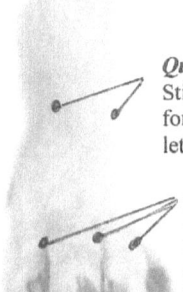

Quartz
Stimulation points
for overweight &
lethargic animals

Amazonite
Release points
for animals
suffering from
hyperactive
fear & stress

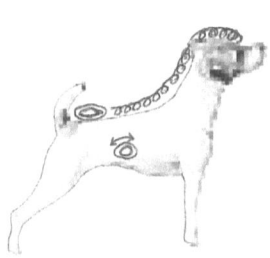

Pass one Teragrams in a clockwise
rotation up the animals spine
from tail to head. Pause where
necessary and allow the neural
spine to balance. The Chakras
will automatically balance. Lastly
Place the pink Teragram on the Spleen
Chakra and rotate in alternative
Clockwise and anticlockwise directions

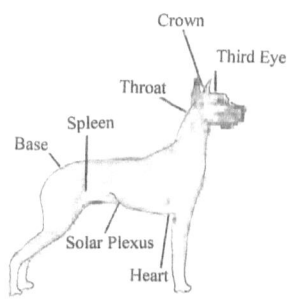

Crown
Third Eye
Throat
Spleen
Base
Solar Plexus
Heart

MAIN CHAKRAS

Products And Services From Sumaris Enterprises

Therapy Kits

Dr. Margaret's Crystal Acupuncture^{sm} Therapy Kit

This amazing set contains 8 crystals and 3 pendulums attractively packaged in a satin purse which can be easily carried in a handbag or pocket. Included in the kit is a Crystal Acupuncture^{sm} booklet. This clear and detailed work gives directions on the use of the points and pendulums and also presents valuable information on the Chakras, the Five Bodies and the acupuncture meridians.

Dr. Margaret's Teragram^{sm} Therapy Kit

Dispel the Madness with our kit containing one each of Natural, Blue, Violet, Red, Green and Pink Agate plates attractively contained in a satin drawstring pouch. A simple instruction booklet provides directions and tips. As a special bonus, we include a CD by Dr. Margaret Rogers Van Coops with a color meditation and a meditation for Chakra and Five Bodies balancing.

Dr. Margaret's "Core" Teragram^{sm} Therapy Kit

Releases Negative History stored in your body's cells. Banishes effects of old issues. Strengthens you to deal with emotional and mental issues. Stimulates more efficient energy flow. Generates inner sense of well-being. Dr.

Margaret's *"Core" Teragram℠ Therapy Kit* contains 3 specially selected Agate slices with a Basic Relaxation Meditation CD featuring the nurturing voice of Dr. Stephen Van Coops. You will quickly enter into a deep alpha state ideal for releasing old emotional habits and irrelevant mind conditioning.

Dr. Margaret's Spiritual Crystal Acupuncture℠ Kit

Five small triangular stones combined with four specially selected pointed stones to refine dense energy and to redirect it according to your desire or need. Kit includes detailed booklet with instructions and diagrams. Spiritual Geometry leads to focus on Spiritual reality beyond your previous physical awareness.

Dr. Margaret's TrinityStone℠ Healing Kit

This unique kit allows auditory memory to stimulate and shift negativity from the body. The five specially selected large open equilateral triangles are used on the Chakras, one at a time, and then all together to erase fear and illusions stored in associations with sounds. Each triangle, when added, will enhance your perception, vision and positive sensations. Included is a booklet with instructions and diagrams and two Serpentine isosceles triangles that are useful in raising the Kundalini and stimulating and harmonizing the Higher and Lower Sacred Centers. When all seven triangles are used together, an awakening may be realized that will result in an explosion of self-confidence.

Books

Breakthrough Therapies:
Crystal Acupuncture℠ & Teragram℠ Therapy

While most people today vaguely realize that the body is a working machine that generates energy, most of us don't understand the way that energy flows, where it goes, and what it does. ***Breakthrough Therapies: Book of Crystal Acupuncture℠ & Teragram℠ Therapy*** is the product of Dr. Margaret's research with her clients and under medical supervision. Her research has validated the integration of the energies of The Five Bodies. The book reveals how the principles of Oriental Acupuncture, combined with the use of specially cut crystals and semi-precious stones, will unblock energy flow in our Five Bodies and will tone, stimulate and balance the Chi energies. Using natural resonating energy stones and crystals such as, but not limited to Hematite, Jasper, Citrine, Amethyst, Carnelian and Quartz, has opened the door to drug-free, inexpensive solutions to emotional and psychological issues ranging from addictions to depression to stress. Dr. Margaret's powerful, non-invasive healing methods also provide remarkable relief from minor physical ailments like headaches to major illnesses and syndromes such as AIDS, Cancer and Multiple Sclerosis. AuthorHouse Publishing Co.

The Book of Crystal Acupuncture^{sm} & Teragram^{sm} Therapy Diagrams

Complementary Healing Therapy has taken another step forward with this amazing book illustrating and describing dozens of crystal stones and tools with techniques for effectively treating acute and chronic conditions suffered by humans and animals. From headaches and minor injuries to major complicated illnesses, Dr. Margaret's treatments provide effective non-invasive and inexpensive remedies to put you or your clients back into a state of positive healing. Dr. Margaret's work with her clients has further validated ancient Oriental Acupuncture principles and merged them with exciting, simple methods using crystals to unblock energy flow in your Five Bodies to tone, balance and stimulate your Chi energies. Her research has carried this work into the treatment of pets and even wildlife. AuthorHouse Publishing Co.

The Way to Oneness

This inspiring work delves into the cosmology of multi-dimensional spiritual existence. Beginning with the "Word" as vibrational consciousness, this book takes you on a journey through the principles of creation, separation, the descending and ascending currents, faith, intuition, belief and evolution. The various sub-divisional cosmologies of the seven archetypes and planes of existence are viewed. Also, incarnation, reincarnation and the Akashic Records are explained as an inter-relationship with the deep subconscious and the Chakras. Of particularly unique interest is the principle of soul fragmentation that the book discusses throughout the text. *The Way to Oneness* concludes with practical steps and techniques for emotional balancing and relaxation, disciplinary exercises and various other psychic tools such as astrology, numerology, graphology and palmistry. Recommended for all practitioners seeking insight into higher knowledge

-- *James Ravenscroft, Whole Life Times March 15. 1990*

The Rejection Syndrome

In our daily lives, all of us experience moments of rejection that create an internal impasse, either by ourselves or by others. My intent is to assist those wishing to be free of those encumbrances brought about by *The Rejection Syndrome*. This is about a pattern of existence that compounds habit, routine and conditioning, leading to limitation, restriction, judgment and competition. Learn about the soul structure and how you can use it to be aware of yourself and to perform to the best of your ability without negativity or rejection. AuthorHouse Publishing Co.

50 Spiritually Powerful Meditations

In the stillness of the mind lies the answer to your purpose. Dr. Margaret has tested all of these meditations herself. By doing each of these meditations, you can find true direction for your life and release fears, pains, restrictions and anger acquired through conditioning. These meditations work! Develop your psychic ability, fine tune your healing skills, mend relationships, empower yourself and much more. This should be a book on everyone's shelf. Jaico Publishing

Pro-Life, Pro-Choice, Pro-Spirit

Spirit's truth is clearly shown through Margaret's own personal experiences. Is everything pre-ordained? The word "abortion" evokes emotions in almost all normally rational minds. Right or wrong? Moral or immoral? Should it be legal or illegal? One of the most burning issues of our time: Advocates of both sides have thrown themselves at each other's faces even to the point of violence. This book is a must read for women who have been, are now or are likely to become pregnant. Without being judgmental, Dr. Margaret provides the wisdom of Master Teachers to assist women to acknowledge, accept and deal with their circumstances. She has crossed the worldly boundaries to discover just what really happens from the point of view of the child-to-be's spirit and spirit Master Teachers. AuthorHouse Publishing Co.

Henry's Secrets

In this gripping mystery, Dr. Margaret Rogers Van Coops, makes her debut into the world of fiction to explore human psyche. Meryl Jones, an African-American single mother has established herself in the world of advertising. Upon the death of her mentor, Henry Wiggins, she is plunged into a stream of events and revelations that turn her world upside down. The story careens into a surprising climax...a web of secrets spills out, changing everyone's lives forever...

Expanding Images

This book fully explains the many aspects of the Psychic Abilities. Through understanding Psychometry, Clairvoyance, Clairaudience and Clairsentience (smell and Taste), with practice on the focus of images, sounds and feelings one can be guided to understand the way to develop these skills and to become a practicing psychic. This book also includes a simple collection of pictorial images of every part of the *OmniCard*tm, where in-depth descriptions of the meanings of these symbols are explained.

Discover Your Baby's Spirit
A Mother's Guide

Every child is joined to its mother before birth through the power of their individual Soul Structures and their earthly personalities. At this time, the Hero, Star, Indigo, Crystal and Liquid Crystal Children are being born.

Dr. Margaret shares how to avoid negative influences while caring for these enlightened children, as well as how to integrate a mother's lifestyle with that of her child from before conception, through birth and into adulthood.

Dr. Margaret has produced an amazing book that will take the reader right into the heart of a mother and her baby. The information is current and thought provoking, and this will help clarify why women choose to be mothers.

Don't miss this opportunity to discover who a child truly is, what their character and destiny might likely be, and to get a glimpse of the wonderful reasons for sharing oneself as a mother. This fascinating work provides simple and clear directions for you to recognize not only the Soul Structures of your family members, but of your own self.

In addition to paperback editions available from this website, "Discover Your Baby's Spirit" is available in electronic formats, including Kindle, from Amazon.com.

Focusing Tool

The OmniCard™

The *OmniCard™* is the simplest way of doing a psychic reading for yourself, your friends or your clients. This revolutionary tool lets you easily tap into images that apply to the question being asked. This can be a wonderful new adventure in learning and psychic awareness. Simply attune to a question and then let your eyes scan the images until one looms up at you. Visualize the significance of the image and all of the meanings it draws forth. It's like having an entire Tarot deck of cards in one stylistic full-color painting, which evokes vivid, literal and symbolic images. These images are the focal points for you to create a psychic reading that will entertain and amaze your friends and clients. Try closing your eyes and letting your hand move over the *OmniCard™*. Your fingers may point to some image of interest or significance. There are many ways to interpret the answers to questions. Try experimenting with them and discover how effective you can be. Special bonus! We are including **Expanding Images,** a special book and glossary of symbols with your *OmniCard™* that will make it even easier for you to match the pictures with their meanings.

Educational Tools

Audio Cd's

Dr. Margaret Rogers Van Coops has given many informative and interesting lectures, which are available on audio CD's. She also provides hypnosis and meditation CD's for focus on specific problems, issues and conditions. Please contact Sumaris Enterprises for titles and prices.

Personal Services

Dr. Margaret is available for private consultations and is also available to do recorded readings by mail or over the phone. Call: (928) 453-7974

Sumaris Enterprises
321 Farallon Dr., Lake Havasu City, AZ 86403, USA.
Website: www.sumariscenter.com
e-mail: drmargaretrvc@gmail.com

ABOUT THE AUTHOR

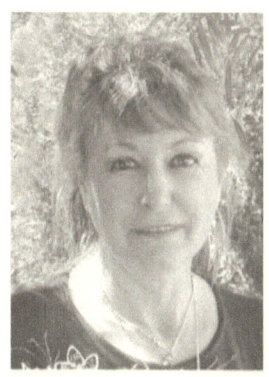 Dr. Margaret Rogers Van Coops has been an ordained minister and missionary of the Universal Christ Church (School of Spiritualism) since 1983. She is currently the Director of Education and Treasurer for UCC. Margaret is a Ph.D. specializing in Medical and Clinical Hypnotherapy and Behavioral Sciences. She is also a DCH(IM), a Doctor of Clinical Hypnotherapy and Integrated Medicine. She has practiced successfully in Spain, France, Switzerland, India, Egypt, Japan, England, Mexico and the United States. Her professional affiliations include the Spiritualist Association of Great Britain, the British Astrological and Psychic Society, The International Medical and Dental Hypnosis Association, the International Association of Counselors and Therapists, the International Hypnosis Federation, the Professional Board of Hypnotherapy and The American Counseling Association. Margaret was among the co-founders of the International Psychic Forum and the American Metaphysical Society. Her dynamic lectures and workshops in Japan and the U.S. have led to regular invitations to speak and participate in international events, including Whole Life Expos and Lifeways/BMSE Expos in various American Cities and The Festivals for Mind, Body and spirit in London and Los Angeles.

She is the author of six other metaphysically oriented texts, including *The Way to Oneness, The Rejection Syndrome, 50 Spiritually Powerful Meditations, Pro-Life, Pro-Choice, Pro Spirit, Breakthrough Therapies: Crystal Acupuncture & Teragram Therapy, The Book of Crystal Acupuncture and*

Teragram Therapy Diagrams and Expanding Images. She has authored two novels: *Regenesis* and *Henry's Secrets.* Her books have been published in Western and Eastern Europe as well as Russia, China, Mexico and India. Dr. Margaret has written screenplays including *The Regenesis Trilogy, Seeing Blind* and *The Survivor,* and she is negotiating production of several reality TV series treatments. Margaret's TV series, Psychic Chit Chat, has been aired weekly on many public access channels in Southern California and Arizona. The show features Dr. Margaret and her husband, Dr. Stephen Van Coops, also a Metaphysician and collaborator on her works.